Study Guide to Accompany

Clinical Drug Therapy

RATIONALES FOR NURSING PRACTICE

Study Guide to Accompany

Clinical Drug Therapy

RATIONALES FOR NURSING PRACTICE

SIXTH EDITION

Gail Ropelewski-Ryan, RN, MSN (Professor)
Nurse Education, Health, Physical Education and Recreation
Corning Community College
Corning, New York

 Lippincott
Philadelphia · New York · Baltimore

Ancillary Editor:	Doris S. Wray
Project Editor:	Debra Schiff
Senior Production Manager:	Helen Ewan
Production Coordinator:	Patricia McCloskey
Art Director:	Carolyn O'Brien
Manufacturing Manager:	William Alberti

9 8 7 6 5 4 3 2 1

ISBN: 0-7817-2401-5

Introduction

The *Study Guide to Accompany Clinical Drug Therapy: Rationales for Nursing Practice,* sixth edition, has been developed to complement Anne Abrams' text. It provides a wealth of learning opportunities to reinforce content that students have read in the text and to promote their ability to apply this information in the patient care setting.

Pharmacology is a tough and demanding science, fraught with seemingly limitless detail about an ever-growing number of drugs. Helping students learn the principles of pharmacology as applied to nursing practice to foster safe and effective management of drug therapy is perhaps one of the most challenging tasks surrounding nursing education today.

The *Study Guide* offers a variety of activities that incorporate approaches to learning designed to accommodate many student learning styles and increase the appeal of learning. The exercises have been chosen to help students establish a connection between how a drug works and why it is used for a particular disorder.

The *Study Guide* will help prepare students in the following ways:

- *Prepare for NCLEX test-taking*:
  NCLEX-style multiple-choice questions in every chapter give students an opportunity to practice their test-taking skills.
- *Develop critical thinking skills*:
  Case study exercises challenge students to develop their critical thinking skills and help students explore how they would apply those skills in a clinical situation.
- *Develop insight about client teaching needs*:
  Each exercise is aimed at expanding the students' knowledge base and understanding of drug therapy and increasing students' understanding of what patients need to know to maximize their drug therapy. Students will use information from the text to develop a teaching plan for persons who will require medication when they return home.
- *Receive immediate reinforcement of learning*:
  Answers for the multiple-choice questions and exercises are provided in the back of the workbook, allowing immediate feedback about the correctness of exercise answers.
- *Expand personal understanding of drug therapy*:
  Completing the exercises and working through the case studies provides valuable opportunity for students to immediately enhance learning effectiveness, building on classroom lectures, textbook reading and reflection, and completion of exercises provided at the end of each text chapter.

Contents

1 Introduction to Pharmacology 1

2 Basic Concepts and Processes 4

3 Administering Medications 7

4 Nursing Process in Drug Therapy 11

5 Physiology of the Central Nervous System 15

6 Opioid Analgesics and Opioid Antagonists 18

7 Analgesic–Antipyretic—
Anti-inflammatory and Related Drugs 21

8 Antianxiety and Sedative-Hypnotic Drugs 24

9 Antipsychotic Drugs 27

10 Antidepressants 32

11 Antiseizure Drugs 36

12 Antiparkinson Drugs 40

13 Skeletal Muscle Relaxants 43

14 Anesthetics 46

15 Substance Abuse Disorders 50

16 Central Nervous System Stimulants 54

17 Physiology of the Autonomic
Nervous System 56

18 Adrenergic Drugs 58

19 Antiadrenergic Drugs 61

20 Cholinergic Drugs 65

21 Anticholinergic Drugs 68

22 Physiology of the Endocrine System 72

23 Hypothalamic and Pituitary Hormones 74

24 Corticosteroids 78

25 Thyroid and Antithyroid Drugs 82

26 Hormones That Regulate Calcium and Bone
Metabolism 86

27 Antidiabetic Drugs 89

28 Estrogens, Progestins, and Oral
Contraceptives 93

29 Androgens and Anabolic Steroids 96

30 Nutritional Support Products and Drugs
for Obesity 99

31 Vitamins 103

32 Minerals and Electrolytes 106

33 General Characteristics of Antimicrobial
Drugs 109

34 Beta-Lactam Antibacterials:
Penicillins, Cephalosporins, and Others 111

35 Aminoglycosides and Fluoroquinolones 114

36 Tetracyclines, Sulfonamides,
and Urinary Agents 117

37 Macrolides and Miscellaneous
Antibacterials 120

38 Drugs for Tuberculosis and *Mycobacterium
Avium* Complex (MAC) Disease 123

39 Antiviral Drugs 126

40 Antifungal Drugs 129

41 Antiparasitics 132

42 Physiology of the Immune System 134

43 Immunizing Agents 136

44 Hematopoietic and Immunostimulant Drugs 140

45 Immunosuppressants 143

46 Physiology of the Respiratory System 146

47 Bronchodilating and Other Antiasthmatic
Drugs 149

48 Antihistamines 152

49 Nasal Decongestants, Antitussives,
Mucolytics, and Cold Remedies 155

50 Physiology of the Cardiovascular System 158

51 Drug Therapy of Heart Failure 161

52 Antiarrhythmic Drugs 165

53 Antianginal Drugs 170

54 Drugs Used in Hypotension and Shock 174

55 Antihypertensive Drugs 177

56 Diuretics 180

57 Drugs That Affect Blood Coagulation 184

58 Drugs for Hyperlipidemia 187

59 Physiology of the Digestive System 189

60 Drugs Used in Peptic Ulcer Disease 192

61 Laxatives and Cathartics 196

62 Antidiarrheals 199

63 Antiemetics 202

64 Drugs Used in Oncologic Disorders 205

65 Drugs Used in Ophthalmic Conditions 209

66 Drugs Used in Dermatologic Conditions 213

67 Drug Use During Pregnancy and Lactation 216

Comprehensive Critical Thinking Exercises 219

Appendix 223

Answers 227

CHAPTER 1

Introduction to Pharmacology

■ Matching Exercise

TERMS AND CONCEPTS

Match the concept with the term for it.

1. _____ The study of drugs.

2. _____ An individual drug that represents a group of drugs.

3. _____ Chemicals that change functions of living organisms.

4. _____ A group of drugs with common characteristics or uses.

5. _____ The law which regulates distribution of opioids and other drugs of abuse.

6. _____ Studies to determine potential uses and adverse effects.

7. _____ A chemical mediator.

8. _____ Related to the chemical name; often indicates the drug group.

9. _____ Designated by the manufacturer.

10. _____ There is an increased number during allergic reactions.

11. _____ The first federal law which established standards for drug products.

12. _____ An important mechanism for transporting protein into cells.

13. _____ A mechanism for secreting intracellular substances into extracellular spaces.

14. _____ An adverse effect involving the liver.

15. _____ Results in edema and impaired cellular function.

A. Drugs

B. Controlled Substances Act

C. Eosinophils

D. Pharmacology

E. Prototype

F. Generic name

G. Drug classification

H. Trade name

I. Histamine

J. Pure Food and Drug Act

K. Clinical trials

L. Exocytosis

M. Hepatotoxicity

N. Cellular injury

O. Pinocytosis

FIGURE 1-1

1. _____
2. _____
3. _____
4. _____
5. _____
6. _____
7. _____
8. _____
9. _____

■ Fill in the Blanks

CELL PHYSIOLOGY, PART I

Fill in the blanks in Figure 1-1 with the terms below.

Golgi apparatus   Cell membrane
Cytoplasm   Mitochondria
Endoplasmic reticulum   Chromatin
Nucleus   Lysosomes
Ribosomes

CELL PHYSIOLOGY, PART II

1. Explain the relationship between the physiology of a body cell and the pharmacodynamics of a drug.

   _____

   _____

2. Examine the role of histamine and prostaglandin in the inflammatory process. _____

   _____

   _____

SOURCES OF DRUGS

1. Historically drugs were derived from

   a. _____

   b. _____

   c. _____

2. Today most drugs are:

   a. _____

■ Review Questions

1. The chemical name given to a drug that is independent of the manufacturer who holds the patent.
   a. Generic name
   b. Brand name
   c. Trade name
   d. Family name

2. Inflammation results in
   a. vasodilation.
   b. cellular damage.
   c. decreased capillary permeability.
   d. decreased blood supply to the injured area.

3. A molecule that, when manipulated, produces a genetically identical molecule is referred to as a
   a. clone.
   b. gene.
   c. hybrid.
   d. encoded protein.

4. Hormones and other substances are produced by the
   a. mitochondria.
   b. cytoplasm.
   c. endoplasmic reticulum.
   d. Golgi complex.

5. The fastest and most effective route of administration for antibiotics is
   a. oral.
   b. subcutaneous.
   c. intravenous.
   d. intramuscular.

6. The standard by which other drugs within a classification are compared.
   a. Prototype
   b. Provisional model
   c. Proximal model
   d. Prototroph

7. The following medication has been transferred from prescription to nonprescription status:
   a. Cimetidine (Tagamet)
   b. Acetaminophen (Tylenol)
   c. Codeine
   d. Diazepam (Valium)

8. The body's main defense against pathogenic bacteria is a group of leukocytes called
   a. nongranulocytes.
   b. basophils.
   c. eosinophils.
   d. neutrophils.

9. Nutrients are broken down by
   a. bradykinin.
   b. enzymes.
   c. exocytosis.
   d. kinins.

10. The following is true regarding drug distribution.
    a. Most drugs in the serum are bound to hormones.
    b. Adequate perfusion is necessary for drug distribution.
    c. Decreased cardiac output increases drug concentration.
    d. Drugs cross the placenta by active transport.

CHAPTER 2

Basic Concepts and Processes

■ Fill in the Blanks

Complete the following sentences.

1. Drug movement and drug action are affected by a drug's ability to _____.

2. _____ soluble drugs cross cell membranes more easily than _____ soluble drugs.

3. _____ is a major determinant of a drug's bioavailability.

4. For most drugs, the presence of food in the stomach _____ the rate of absorption.

5. Besides the stomach, other absorptive sites include _____ and _____.

6. Distribution depends largely on the _____.

7. An important factor in drug distribution is _____.

8. Only the free or _____ portion of a drug acts on body cells.

9. The _____ regulates diffusion of drug molecules from the bloodstream into brain tissue.

10. _____ is the method by which drugs are inactivated or biotransformed by the body.

11. Most drugs are metabolized by _____ in the _____.

12. Some drugs stimulate liver cells to produce larger amounts of drug metabolizing enzymes. This is referred to as _____.

13. Organs of excretion include the _____, _____, _____, and _____.

14. Receptors that bind with drugs include _____, _____, and nucleic acids.

15. When molecules bind with receptor molecules, it initiates physiochemical reactions that _____ or _____ cellular function.

16. The _____ available to interact with drug molecules also affects the extent of drug action.

17. A drug's _____ affects its ability to reach tissue fluids.

18. Route of _____ affects drug actions and responses by influencing _____ and _____.

19. Drug actions may be more pronounced in _____, _____, and older adults because of their _____ and _____ function.

20. Cross tolerance is attributed to _____.

■ Definitions

Define each of the following terms.

1. Passive diffusion

   _____

   _____

   _____

2. Active transport

   _____

   _____

   _____

3. Excretion

   _____

   _____

   _____

4. Serum half-life

   _____

   _____

   _____

5. Agonists

   _____

   _____

   _____

6. Antagonists

   _____

   _____

   _____

7. Synergism

   _____

   _____

   _____

8. Idiosyncrasy

   _____

   _____

   _____

9. Enzyme induction

   _____

   _____

   _____

10. Drug fever

   _____

   _____

   _____

■ Matching Exercise

TERMS AND CONCEPTS

Match the concept with the term for it.

1. _____ Food ingested with oral medications

2. _____ Coumadin

3. _____ MAO inhibitor

4. _____ Tetracycline

A. Combines with calcium in milk to form an insoluble compound.

B. Slows absorption and gastric emptying.

C. Food high in vitamin K will decrease its effect.

D. Ingestion of food high in tyramine and this drug can cause hypertension.

■ Review Questions

1. When reviewing the product information available on a drug, the nurse finds that the drug is teratogenic. The nurse would know that this drug should not be administered to

   a. asthmatic clients.

   b. pregnant clients.

   c. children.

   d. clients with renal failure.

2. Taking erythromycin with food will

   a. enhance the rate of absorption.

   b. prolong the therapeutic effect.

   c. decrease the rate of elimination.

   d. delay the rate of absorption.

3. Following a diagnosis of meningitis, the physician ordered penicillin G for your client. This drug was selected because it is

   a. fat soluble and able to cross the blood–brain barrier.

   b. water soluble and crosses the blood–brain barrier in the presence of inflammation.

   c. transported to the brain via active transport.

   d. one of the few drugs that uses passive diffusion to reach the brain.

4. You admit a chronic alcoholic with Crohn's disease and peripheral edema who smokes two packs of cigarettes a day. You will assess him for possible toxic drug effects primarily related to

   a. decreased lung capacity.

   b. impaired liver function.

   c. decreased cardiac output.

   d. impaired absorption.

5. Your client, who has been using nitroglycerin for 5 years, complains that it does not work as it used to. This is an example of

   a. supersensitivity.

   b. an agonist response.

   c. tolerance.

   d. an idiosyncrasy.

6. Your client's lab work indicates hypoalbuminemia. This can result in

   a. decreased drug metabolism.

   b. prolonged half-life of a medication.

   c. excess free drug and an exaggerated effect.

   d. a reduced therapeutic effect.

7. Your client is to be started on warfarin (Coumadin). She has been taking aspirin daily for arthritis for 5 years. You notify her physician of this because

   a. aspirin increases platelet aggregation.

   b. aspirin displaces Coumadin from the binding site, increasing bleeding potential.

   c. aspirin creates an acidic environment, which inhibits Coumadin absorption.

   d. Coumadin administered with aspirin results in excessive clotting.

8. Which of the following statements is true regarding the half-life of medications?

   a. Increasing the dose will increase the half-life of the medication.

   b. Five half-lives are usually required for a medication to be completely excreted.

   c. Clients with renal disease usually have decreased drug half-lives.

   d. The half-life of a drug determines how often the drug is to be administered.

9. All of the following will affect a client's response to medications except

   a. psychological state.

   b. climate.

   c. body weight.

   d. age.

10. Your client, who is being treated with a MAO inhibitor for depression, ate aged cheese and wine for dinner. She will likely have the following response:

    a. severe headache.

    b. diarrhea.

    c. decreased urinary output.

    d. no ill effects.

CHAPTER 3

Administering Medications

■ Matching Exercise

TERMS AND CONCEPTS

Match the concept with the term for it.

1. _____ An acceptable site for IM injections.

2. _____ Both eyes.

3. _____ Narcotic analgesics and other drugs with potential for abuse.

4. _____ One ounce.

5. _____ Before meals.

6. _____ Units of measurements in the metric system.

7. _____ IV, IM, SC injections.

8. _____ Glass containers that may contain one or several doses.

9. _____ An acceptable site for SC injections.

10. _____ Under the tongue.

11. _____ Glass containers that contain approximately one dose of a drug.

12. _____ The vastus lateralis muscle is a commonly used location for IM injection in this group.

13. _____ An anatomic landmark for administering an injection in the deltoid muscle.

14. _____ A drug preparation suitable for use in the eye.

15. _____ A dosage form designed to dissolve in the small intestine rather than in the stomach.

16. _____ A drug preparation suitable for use in the ear.

17. _____ Applied to the skin.

18. _____ Administration of this medication requires the use of a special syringe.

19. _____ Physicians administer medication in this location.

20. _____ A suppository can be administered here.

A. Controlled drugs

B. Ventrogluteal

C. 30 mL

D. a.c.

E. Meter, gram, liter

F. OU

G. Parenteral

H. Vials

I. Abdomen

J. Sublingual

K. Topical

L. Ampules

M. Acromion process

N. Ophthalmic solution

O. Children

P. Enteric coated

Q. 240 mL

R. Otic

S. Insulin

T. Demerol

U. Intrathecal

V. Intravaginally

ABBREVIATIONS

Match each abbreviation (numbered items) with its defin-
ition (lettered items). Each definition may be used only
once.

1. _____ q.d.
2. _____ PRN
3. _____ q.i.d.
4. _____ stat
5. _____ qlh
6. _____ h.s.
7. _____ IM
8. _____ SL
9. _____ PO
10. _____ OU

A. Both eyes
B. Intramuscular
C. Immediately
D. Sublingual
E. Bedtime
F. When needed
G. Four times daily
H. Oral
I. Once daily
J. Every hour

EQUIVALENTS

Match each quantity (numbered items) with its equivalent
(lettered items). Each equivalent may be used only once.

1. _____ 0.6 g
2. _____ 60, 64, or 65 mg
3. _____ 1000 mL
4. _____ 8 oz
5. _____ 300 mg
6. _____ 650 mg
7. _____ 30 mL
8. _____ 5 mL
9. _____ 2.2 lb
10. _____ 1 L

A. 0.3 g
B. 30 cc
C. 1 gr
D. 10 gr
E. 600 mg
F. 1 tsp
G. 1 kg
H. 1 L
I. 1 lb
J. 1 tbsp
K. 250 mL
L. 1 quart

■ Diagram

SUBCUTANEOUS INJECTIONS

Mark on Figure 3-1 where subcutaneous injections can be
administered.

FIGURE 3-1

■ Practice Questions

MEDICATION ORDERS

1. The physician's order reads: Administer ASA p.c. What time will you give the medication?
   a. 10 PM
   b. 9 AM
   c. 8 AM, 1 PM, 6 PM
   d. 7 AM, 11 AM, 4 PM

2. The physician's order reads: Administer Maalox at a.c. and h.s. When will you administer the medication?
   a. 7 AM, 11 AM, 4 PM, 9 PM
   b. 9 AM, 9 PM
   c. 10 AM, 2 PM, 6 PM, 10 PM
   d. 7 AM, 7 PM

3. The physician's order reads: Administer furosemide (Lasix) b.i.d. You will administer it
   a. daily.
   b. every other day.
   c. twice a day.
   d. on odd days.

■ Dosage Calculations

PRACTICE SET I

1. Order: Ferrous sulfate 600 mg PO.
   Label: Ferrous sulfate 325 mg/tablet.
   Administer:

   _____

2. Order: Penicillin 250,000 units IV.
   Label: Penicillin 20 million units in 20 mL.
   Administer:

   _____

3. Order: KCl 40 mEq PO.
   Label: KCl 10 mEq/15 mL.
   Administer:

   _____

4. Order: Digoxin 0.375 mg PO.
   Label: Digoxin 0.125 mg/tablet.
   Administer:

   _____

5. Order: Atropine 0.2 mg IM.
   Label: Atropine 0.4 mg/cc.
   Administer:

   _____

6. Order: Demerol 30 mg IM.
   Label: Demerol 75 mg/cc.
   Administer:

   _____

7. Order: Gentamicin 50 mg IV.
   Label: Gentamicin 80 mg/2 mL.
   Administer:

   _____

8. Order: Aminophylline 0.4 g IV.
   Label: Aminophylline 500 mg/10 cc.
   Administer:

   _____

9. Order: Heparin 4000 units IV.
   Label: Heparin 1000 unit/mL.
   Administer:

   _____

10. Order: Digoxin 0.125 mg IM.
    Label: Digoxin 0.5 mg/2 cc.
    Administer:

    _____

PRACTICE SET II

1. Two ounces are equivalent to how many milliliters? _____

2. The physician writes an order for 1 gram of aspirin. Each tablet contains 5 grains. How many tablets will you administer? _____

3. Mr. J. is to receive 12 ounces of magnesium citrate. How many milliliters should he receive?
   _____

4. Mr. P. weighs 132 lb. How many kilograms does he weigh? _____

5. You want Mrs. S. to drink 1.25 liters of solution. How many milliliters is she expected to drink?
   _____

6. The physician writes an order for 125 mg. The bottle is marked 50 mg/mL. How many milliliters will you administer? _____

7. The order reads "administer 20 grains." On hand you have grams. How many grams will you administer? _____

8. An ampule contains 50 mg of a drug in 2 mL of solution. The physician orders 10 mg of the drug. How many milliliters will you administer? _____

9. The order reads "administer 2500 units of heparin SC." The vial contains 10,000 units/mL. How many milliliters will you administer? _____

10. The order reads "give 10 mL" of a solution. Mrs. J. wants to know how many teaspoons or tablespoons this equals. The best answer would be _____.

■ Review Questions

DOSAGE CALCULATIONS

1. Order: Aspirin 5 gr PO.
   Label: Aspirin 325 mg/tablet.
   Administer
   a. 1 tablet.
   b. 1½ tablet.
   c. 2 tablets.
   d. 2½ tablets.

2. Order: Penicillin 500,000 units IV.
   Label: Penicillin 20 million units in 20 mL.
   Administer
   a. 0.5 mL.
   b. 1 mL.
   c. 1.5 mL.
   d. 2 mL.

3. Order: KCl 20 mEq PO.
   Label: KCl 10 mEq/15 mL.
   Administer
   a. 10 mL.
   b. 15 mL.
   c. 20 mL.
   d. 30 mL.

4. Order: Digoxin 0.25 mg PO.
   Label: Digoxin 0.125 mg/tablet.
   Administer
   a. 1 tablet.
   b. 2 tablets.
   c. 4 tablets.
   d. 5 tablets.

5. Order: Atropine 0.6 mg IM.
   Label: Atropine 0.4 mg/cc.
   Administer
   a. 0.75 cc.
   b. 1.25 cc.
   c. 1.50 cc.
   d. 1.75 cc.

6. Order: Demerol 30 mg IM.
   Label: Demerol 100 mg/cc.
   Administer
   a. 0.3 cc.
   b. 0.4 cc.
   c. 0.5 cc.
   d. 0.6 cc.

7. Order: Heparin 2500 units SC.
   Label: Heparin 10,000 units/mL.
   Administer
   a. 0.25 mL.
   b. 0.5 mL.
   c. 0.75 mL.
   d. 1 mL.

8. Order: Gentamicin 65 mg IV.
   Label: Gentamicin 80 mg/2 mL.
   Administer
   a. 1.5 mL.
   b. 1.6 mL.
   c. 1.3 mL.
   d. 1.4 mL.

9. Order: Aminophylline 0.5 g IV.
   Label: Aminophylline 500 mg/10 cc.
   Administer
   a. 1 cc.
   b. 10 cc.
   c. 100 cc.
   d. 1000 cc.

10. Order: Heparin 2000 units IV.
    Label: Heparin 1000 unit/mL.
    Administer
    a. 1 mL.
    b. 2 mL.
    c. 3 mL.
    d. 4 mL.

CHAPTER 4

Nursing Process in Drug Therapy

■ True or False

1. _____ When effective, it is generally better to use as few drugs in as low doses as possible.

2. _____ Fixed-dose combinations of two or three drugs are preferred over two or three single drugs, when available.

3. _____ Clients with severe renal disease often need smaller-than-average doses of drugs that are excreted by the kidney.

4. _____ Some drugs can be given safely during pregnancy.

5. _____ The preferred site for IM injection in infants is the thigh.

6. _____ The most accurate method of calculating drug dosages for children is a method based on age.

7. _____ Drug therapy in newborn infants must be very cautious because of immature liver and kidney functions.

8. _____ Adverse drug effects are more likely to occur in elderly clients than in young or middle-aged adults.

9. _____ Newer drugs are more effective than older ones.

10. _____ The nurse should assess the client's condition before giving PRN medications.

11. _____ Drugs with long half-lives may not reach maximum therapeutic effect for several days or weeks.

12. _____ Older adults have decreased amounts of body fat, so fat-soluble drugs have a shorter duration of action.

13. _____ Decreased serum protein levels can result in increased serum concentration and increased risk of adverse effects.

14. _____ When doing a medication history, the nurse should also ask about nonprescription drug use, including alcohol, caffeine, and nicotine.

15. _____ A client's renal function should be considered before drug therapy is started.

■ Critical Thinking Case Study

PEDIATRIC CALCULATIONS

M., a 5-year-old child, is admitted to your unit with a seizure disorder. M. weighs 44 lb. The recommended dosage range of phenobarbital is 4–6 mg/kg/day for anticonvulsant effects.

1. Identify the maximum daily dosage.

2. If the above amount is to be given in three equal doses, what is the amount (mg) per dose?

3. The pharmacy sends you a phenobarbital solution containing 15 mg/mL. How many milliliters are needed for each dose calculated above?

M. is to be started on phenytoin (Dilantin). The recommended dosage range of phenytoin (Dilantin) is 4–7 mg/kg/day. The pharmacy sends a solution of 100 mg/2 mL.

4. Identify the minimum daily dose (mg).

5. Identify the maximum daily dose (mg).

6. You are to administer the maximum daily dose to M. in two equal doses. Identify the amount needed (mL) for each dose.

Display 4-1. Medication History

Name _____ Age _____

Occupation _____ Educational level _____

Health problems, acute and chronic

Do you have any allergies?

If yes, describe specific effects or symptoms.

Part I. Prescription Medications

Do you take any prescription medications on a regular basis? If yes, ask the following about each medication:

Name: _____ Dose: _____

Frequency: _____ Specific times: _____

How long taken: _____

Reason for use: _____

Are you able to take this medicine pretty much as prescribed?

What do you do when you miss a dose of medication?

Does anyone else help you take your medication?

What information or instructions were you given when the medication was first prescribed?

Do you think the medication is doing what it was prescribed to do?

Have you had any problems that you attribute to the medication?

Do you take any prescription medications on an irregular basis?

If yes, ask the following about each medication:

Name: _____ Reason for use: _____

Dose: _____ How long taken: _____

Frequency: _____

Part II. Nonprescription Medications

Do you take any OTC medications for the following problems?

Problem	Yes/No	Medication Name	Amount	Frequency
Pain				
Headache				
Sleep				
Cold				
Indigestion				
Heartburn				
Diarrhea				
Constipation				
Other				

Part III. Social Habits

	Yes/No	Amount
Coffee (decaffeinated, regular)		
Tea (decaffeinated, regular)		
Soda (decaffeinated, regular, sugar-free)		
Alcohol		
Tobacco		
Candy (chocolates, licorice, diet candy)		

Part IV. Physicians

Name	What You Are Seeing Them For	Phone
_____	_____	_____
_____	_____	_____
_____	_____	_____

M. is complaining of pain. The physician orders 6 mg of morphine subcutaneously q6h. The recommended dosage range of morphine for a child is 0.1–0.2 mg/kg.

7. Identify where you would administer the medication.

8. Determine whether the dose ordered for M. is acceptable, and discuss what you do.

■ Obtaining a Medication History

Using the form on page 12, select a patient, friend, or family member and obtain his or her medical history.

■ Review Questions

1. A 90-year-old is started on digoxin (Lanoxin); because of the client's age, the dosage of this medication may need to be adjusted due to his
   a. increased body fat.
   b. decreased gastrointestinal secretions.
   c. decreased glomerular filtration rate.
   d. lack of ability to metabolize drugs.

2. A 3-month-old is receiving a topical steroid; because of the increased absorption of topical drugs in infants, you should assess for
   a. increased elimination of other medications.
   b. fluid volume overload.
   c. decreased urinary output.
   d. suppressed adrenal cortical function.

3. The following physiologic characteristic of the elderly may increase the serum concentrations of drugs that are bound to protein:
   a. decreased cardiac output.
   b. decreased serum albumin.
   c. decreased liver enzymes.
   d. decreased number of functioning nephrons.

4. S., age 6, refuses to take her antibiotic. To proceed, you should
   a. hold S. down, open her mouth, and administer the medication.
   b. tell S. you will administer the medication by injection if she does not cooperate.
   c. mix the medication with a favorite food or fluid to make it more acceptable.
   d. call S.'s mother and ask her to come in and assist you.

5. Which of the following statements is true in regard to the administration of water-soluble drugs in infants as compared to adults?
   a. A smaller portion of the infant's body is water; therefore, the infant requires smaller dosages.
   b. A larger portion of the infant's body is water; therefore, the infant requires larger doses of water-soluble drugs.
   c. A smaller portion of the infant's body is fat; therefore, the infant requires a larger dose of water-soluble drugs.
   d. A larger portion of the infant's body is water, but usually a smaller dose is needed.

6. A 75-year-old client has just received an initial dose of lithium. Because of his total body water composition, you would expect that the onset of action of lithium will
   a. be rapid and result in higher plasma concentrations.
   b. take longer and the duration will be prolonged.
   c. be rapid and the duration of action will be cut in half.
   d. be prolonged and result in lower plasma concentrations.

7. Before administering medications to a 9-month-old, the nurse should be aware that his or her decreased capacity for biotransformation of drugs will
   a. reduce blood levels of certain drugs.
   b. slow the metabolism and elimination of certain drugs.
   c. significantly limit the types of medications that can be administered.
   d. decrease the possibility of drug toxicity.

8. When digoxin (Lanoxin) is started, a relatively large dose may be administered. This is referred to as a
    a. therapeutic dose.
    b. loading dose.
    c. maintenance dose.
    d. fixed dose.

9. The percentage of body water of an infant is
    a. 20%–30%.
    b. 30%–40%.
    c. 50%–60%.
    d. 70%–80%.

10. A 4-year-old child, weighing 22.8 kg, is to receive ampicillin (Omnipen). The adult dose is 450 mg q6h. Using Clark's rule [(weight in pounds ÷ 150) x Adult dose = Child dose], determine the appropriate dose.
    a. 100 mg
    b. 150 mg
    c. 200 mg
    d. 250 mg

CHAPTER 5

Physiology of the Central Nervous System

■ Fill in the Blanks

Complete the following sentences.

1. The central nervous system is composed of the
   _____ and _____.

2. Excitability is the _____.

3. Conductivity is the _____.

4. Three types of neurotransmitters are
   _____, _____, and _____.

5. The amines include _____, _____,
   and _____.

6. The cerebral cortex is involved in all
   _____.

7. The thalamus receives impulses carrying sensations
   such as _____, _____,
   _____, and _____.

8. The hypothalamus maintains homeostasis by making continuous adjustments in _____,
   _____, _____,_____,
   _____, and _____.

9. The medulla oblongata contains neurons that form
   the vital _____, _____, and
   _____ centers.

10. When stimulated, the reticular formation produces
    _____ and _____.

11. The limbic system regulates _____,
    _____, _____, and _____.

12. The cerebellum coordinates _____. It also
    helps to maintain _____ and
    _____.

13. Pyramidal tracts carry impulses from the brain to
    the spinal cord to the _____.

14. Extrapyramidal tracts do not enter the
    _____.

15. A lack of oxygen is called _____.

16. Hypoglycemia causes _____,
    _____, _____, _____, and
    _____.

17. _____ is required for the production and
    use of glucose.

18. A thiamine deficiency can cause degeneration of
    the _____ and can lead to _____
    syndrome.

19. Moderate CNS depression produces
    _____, _____, _____, and
    _____.

20. Severe CNS depression produces _____,
    loss of reflexes, _____, and _____.

21. Mild CNS stimulants produce _____,
    _____, and _____.

22. Moderate CNS stimulants produce _____,
    _____, _____, and _____.

23. Excessive CNS stimulation can cause
    _____, _____, and _____.

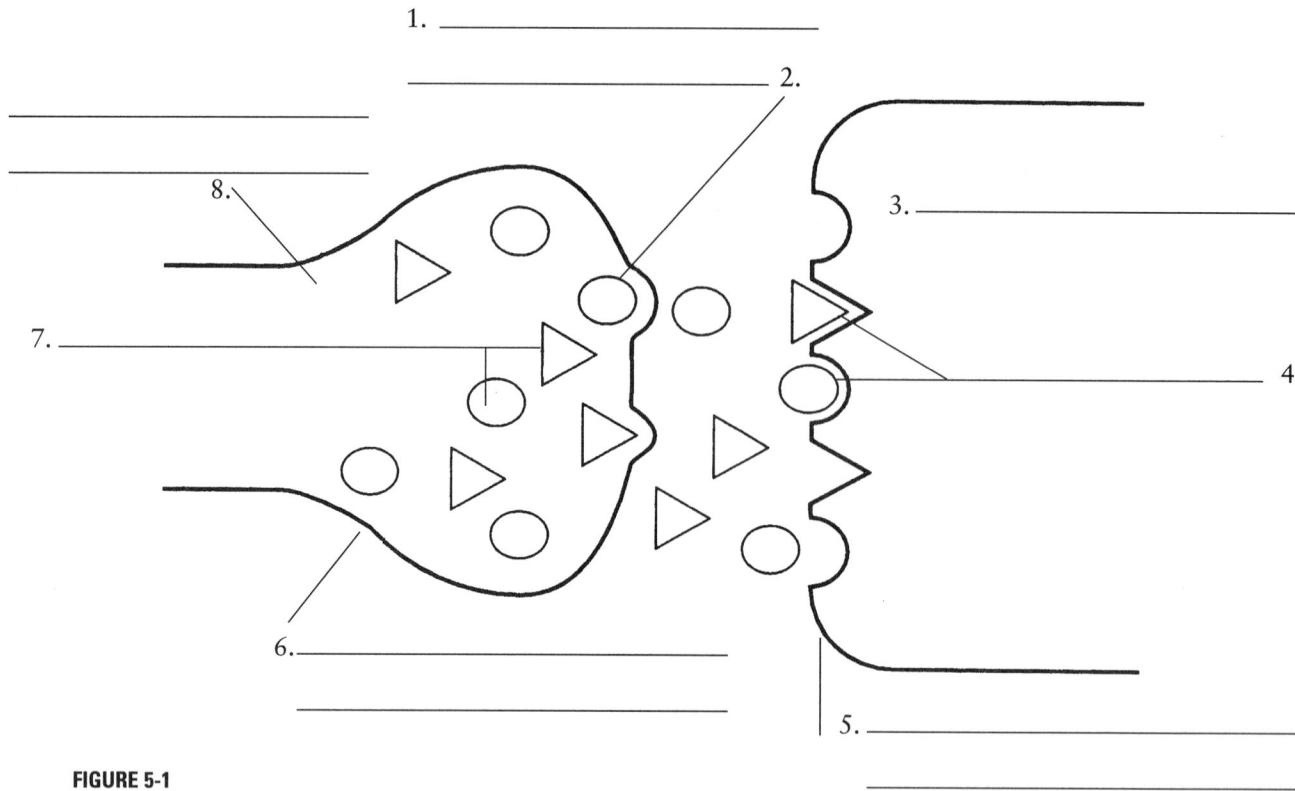

1. _____

2. _____

3. _____

4. _____

5. _____

6. _____

7. _____

8.

FIGURE 5-1

■ Neurotransmission, Part I

Neurotransmitter molecules, released by the presynaptic nerve, cross the synapse and bind with receptor proteins in the cell membrane of the postsynaptic nerve.

Fill in the blanks in Figure 5-1 with the terms below.

Receptor sites
Neurotransmitters
Presynaptic nerve terminal
Presynaptic nerve cell membrane
Postsynaptic nerve terminal
Synapse
Release site
Postsynaptic nerve cell membrane

■ Neurotransmission, Part II

Complete the following sentences.

1. Norepinephrine is an excitatory neurotransmitter that affects mood and motor activity after crossing the _____ from the postganglionic sympathetic nervous system neurons and binding to _____ in the postsynaptic nerve cell membrane of the nerves that supply blood vessels to the adrenal medulla.

2. Acetylcholine is an inhibitory neurotransmitter that exerts inhibitory effects on organs supplied by the vagus nerves by binding at _____.

■ Review Questions

1. Your client has had a cerebrovascular accident (CVA) and he has short-term memory loss. Which part of his brain was affected by the CVA?
   a. Limbic system
   b. Reticular formation network
   c. Cerebral cortex
   d. Cerebellum

2. Glucose is required for
   a. adequate cerebral blood flow.
   b. cell metabolism.
   c. oxygen utilization.
   d. transference of nerve impulses.

3. Lack of dopamine causes Parkinson's disease, which is characterized by
   a. hyperactive reflexes and muscle spasms.
   b. slurred speech and memory loss.
   c. muscle weakness and dizziness.
   d. rigidity and increased muscle tone.

4. Thirst and appetite centers are located in the
   a. thalamus.
   b. cerebellum.
   c. medulla oblongata.
   d. hypothalamus.

5. Mild CNS depression can produce
   a. short attention span.
   b. decreased muscle tone.
   c. decreased perception of sensation.
   d. loss of reflexes.

6. The area of the brain responsible for temperature regulation is the
   a. limbic system.
   b. cerebellum.
   c. medulla oblongata.
   d. hypothalamus.

7. After surgery, Mr. S.'s respiratory rate falls to 10. Which portion of the brain helps to regulate respiration?
   a. Medulla oblongata
   b. Limbic system
   c. Hypothalamus
   d. Cerebrum

8. Severe hypoglycemia can cause
   a. degeneration of the myelin sheath.
   b. encephalopathy.
   c. seizures.
   d. hypotension.

9. After a tumor is removed from the cerebellum, the nurse needs to monitor
   a. muscular coordination.
   b. memory loss.
   c. respiratory depression.
   d. intake and output.

10. Excessive CNS stimulation can cause
    a. insomnia.
    b. excessive talking.
    c. nervousness.
    d. cardiac dysrhythmias.

CHAPTER **6**

Opioid Analgesics and Opioid Antagonists

■ Fill in the Blanks

Complete the following sentences.

1. CNS effects of opioid analgesics include:

   a. _____

   b. _____

   c. _____

   d. _____

   e. _____

2. Opioids affect the GI system by _____ and causing _____.

3. Morphine sulfate can be administered _____, _____, _____, _____, _____, _____, and _____.

4. Roxanol _____/mL and MS Contin _____/tab sustained release have been developed for cancer patients with chronic pain.

5. Fentanyl (Duragesic) may be administered by a _____ and a _____ which lasts _____.

6. Codeine is often given with _____ for additive analgesic effects.

7. Meperidine hydrochloride (Demerol) differs from morphine in that it is _____ and causes _____. The usual dose of meperidine is _____ every _____ hours.

8. Three examples of non-opioid drugs used for moderate to severe pain are _____, _____, and _____.

9. Opioid antagonists used to treat opioid overdoses are _____, _____, and _____.

10. Before administering pain medication you should _____.

11. Specific assessment data usually include _____, _____, _____, and _____.

12. Besides the administration of pain medications, other nursing measures that can be employed include _____, application of _____, and _____ techniques.

13. The _____ route of administration is preferred when administering opioids for acute pain because _____.

14. A _____ allows clients to self-administer pain medication.

15. Two other routes of administration are _____ or _____ and _____.

16. _____ can be used with opioid analgesics for the treatment of various types of colic because it reduces the spasms caused by opioid analgesics.

17. Infants experiencing pain will demonstrate _____, _____, and _____.

18. _____ suppositories are used more often in children.

19. Elderly adults should be monitored for _____ or _____ and _____.

20. Drug doses need to be reduced if the client has _____ impairment.

21. Opioid analgesics may cause _____, _____, _____, and _____.

■ Review Questions

1. Which of the following assessments is the result of administration of opioids?
   a. Tachycardia
   b. Hypertension
   c. Hyperactive bowel sounds
   d. Pupillary constriction

2. When administering morphine, it is important to assess for
   a. respiratory depression.
   b. absent bowel sounds.
   c. bradycardia.
   d. decreased urinary output.

3. An example of an opioid analgesic used for moderate pain is
   a. oxymorphone hydrochloride (Numorphan).
   b. codeine sulfate.
   c. morphine sulfate (Roxanol).
   d. butorphanol tartrate (Stadol).

4. A common side effect of the administration of opiates is
   a. constipation.
   b. bradycardia.
   c. dry mouth.
   d. blurred vision.

5. A physician during World War II ran out of pain medication for his men who had been injured in battle, so he administered normal saline and the men were relieved of their pain. This is an example of
   a. pain threshold.
   b. pain perception.
   c. behavioral response.
   d. placebo response.

6. The drug of choice for pain relief for end-stage cancer patients is
   a. morphine sulfate (Roxanol).
   b. propoxyphene (Darvon).
   c. codeine sulfate.
   d. meperidine hydrochloride (Demerol).

7. Which of the following statements by Mr. C. indicates that he understands the preoperative teaching you have done?
   a. "I will ask for medication every 4 hours whether I need it or not."
   b. "I will take the pain medication so that I will be able to turn, cough, and take a deep breath."
   c. "I will avoid taking the pain medication because it will impair my ability to ambulate and impede my recovery."
   d. "No matter how bad the pain gets, I am not to ask for medication before 4 hours."

8. Pain-relieving substances produced by the body include
   a. opioids.
   b. histamine.
   c. bradykinins.
   d. endorphins.

9. The following medications, if administered concurrently with morphine, may produce hypotension.
   a. Antihistamines
   b. Antidiabetic agents
   c. Thyroid preparations
   d. Diuretics

10. The physician has ordered a PCA (patient-controlled analgesia) pump for Mrs. J. after her abdominal surgery to
    a. relieve the nursing staff of q4h administration of pain medication.
    b. eliminate the administration of IV medications.
    c. provide small amounts of pain medication at regular intervals throughout the day.
    d. reduce the amount of pain medication used.

■ Word Find

Place the trade name (if it exists) next to the generic name, then circle the word in the word find.

1. _____ fentanyl
2. _____ codeine
3. _____ meperidine
4. _____ hydromorphone
5. _____ morphine
6. _____ butorphanol
7. _____ propoxyphene
8. _____ nalbuphine
9. _____ naloxone
10. _____ pentazocine

WORD FIND

```
N O T H S B H Y P O F T I L C L C E F G H H J N K
K A D R E N E R G I C E N B E T A Z O L O L A N E
C M R I A S S A N L L X Q K E Z S V C D N C A T V
X Y Z T I P L D N E D R O N O N I R L A R N V R R
H L P O D I L A U D I D I C A Y Y O D A V V P P J
F N V A N L I C B R E E K X F H T G N A E S O S B
R I L U A A C A I D D U K L O E E U U E T O R R P
X T O S H R F R N O H A Z Y P X D K B B L K A O T
L R N A Y J R E C L N O S T Y H P E A N B E R E C
V A S G O N I Q P F E N T A N Y L K I S N L O K C
X T K X T G A A N G N P A P E C O R N I U O U S A
K J K X C Z A B T N T A D P V C D T E G F G X H O
V A S D I P I O C P R A O Z O I N J K A J K L D N
O N A E S O R P T I O N L W N C I N U C N C I V O
P T O M I I A N G I N Y B W I X K U N L S I N E T
A Z A E Y B I D L E S X F N I N S V D F H I A N I
R S C R F X Z Y N G R H V T G N J N A A E Z H T L
G E M O R P H I N E V K O N M H C H L O R Z I D E
Y N O L G D B P Q E R R O T V S P Q Y L O V B P C
L W I E F I C D L S N E V H O W G Y O Z A J O W D
F D O M R G G L I I S T P R O T E R E N E R Z N X
N C O E U M A D I N S F T P T M I G J F U W T C Y
E F D D Q C N Q N T A T D Y M N S J Z E B G O G C
```

■ Critical Thinking Case Study

M.G., a 29-year-old woman, had a simple mastectomy 3 days ago. She has been receiving 50 mg meperidine hydrochloride (Demerol) IM every 4 hours for pain since returning from surgery. You medicate her with two Tylenol No. 3 at 10:30 AM. Before you help her out of bed, she states, "The Demerol makes me feel so much better. I don't think this medication is going to work."

1. How you would respond to her statement?

2. Describe the adverse effects you are assessing for.

While you are at lunch, M.G. requests Demerol and one of your colleagues administers it.

3. Discuss what you would do when you return from lunch and find out M.G. has been medicated.

CHAPTER 7

Analgesic—Antipyretic— Anti-inflammatory and Related Drugs

■ Matching Exercise

TERMS AND CONCEPTS

Match the concept with the term for it.

1. _____ Toxic doses of this drug can cause liver necrosis.

2. _____ This drug has antiplatelet properties.

3. _____ The normal body response to tissue damage.

4. _____ Substances found in body tissue that help regulate cell function.

5. _____ A drug used in the treatment of gout.

6. _____ A drug used only for the treatment of migraine headaches.

7. _____ An ibuprofen drug available without a prescription.

8. _____ A classic sign of an aspirin overdose.

9. _____ A NSAID effective in the treatment of juvenile arthritis.

10. _____ May be caused by dehydration, infectious process, and brain injury.

A. Inflammation

B. Ergotamine tartrate (Ergomar)

C. Ringing in the ears

D. Acetaminophen (Tylenol)

E. Acetylsalicylic acid (ASA)

F. Naproxen (Naprosyn)

G. Advil

H. Allopurinol (Zyloprim)

I. Prostaglandins

J. Fever

K. Headache

■ True or False

1. _____ Gangrene of the extremities has occurred after the administration of ergotamine tartrate (Ergomar).

2. _____ Therapeutic effects from ergot preparations are usually evident within an hour after the drug is administered.

3. _____ Allopurinol (Zyloprim) is administered for acute attacks of gout.

4. _____ Persons taking indomethacin (Indocin) need to be assessed for confusion and depression.

5. _____ Clients receiving colchicine should be examined frequently for bone marrow depression.

6. _____ Diflunisal (Dolobid) is equal or superior to ASA for arthritis pain.

7. _____ Ketoprofen (Orudis) is better tolerated than ASA but can still cause many of the adverse effects associated with ASA.

8. _____ No anti-inflammatory/analgesic medication can be administered parenterally.

9. _____ Acetaminophen lacks anti-inflammatory and antiplatelet effects.

10. _____ Gastrointestinal problems occur commonly with anti-inflammatory and anti-gout agents.

11. _____ NSAIDs may be given shortly after birth to close a patent ductus arteriosus.

12. _____ Gold may be used to treat rheumatoid arthritis.

■ Review Questions

1. A 29-year-old man admitted with chronic ergot poisoning will be assessed for
   a. neurotoxicity.
   b. renal failure.
   c. hepatotoxicity.
   d. circulatory impairment.

2. Which of the following medications, if administered concurrently with sulfinpyrazone (Anturane), will decrease its effects?
   a. Aspirin
   b. Acetaminophen (Tylenol)
   c. Antidiabetic agents
   d. Maalox

3. A client taking an ergot preparation for a migraine headache should be told to report
   a. nausea and vomiting.
   b. sore throat and fever.
   c. skin rash or upset stomach.
   d. numbness or tingling of the extremities.

4. Which of the following statements by your client indicates that she has understood the teaching that you have done about relief of migraine headaches?
   a. "I will take the medication only after I have tried other remedies."
   b. "After taking the medication, I should get relief of headache pain within 5–10 minutes."
   c. "After I take the medication, I will lie down in a quiet, dark room."
   d. "If I think there is a possibility that I might get a headache, I will take the medication."

5. The drug used in the treatment of gout that lowers uric acid levels is
   a. ibuprofen (Motrin).
   b. allopurinol (Zyloprim).
   c. hydroxychloroquine (Plaquenil).
   d. cyclophosphamide (Cytoxan).

6. Your client is started on indomethacin (Indocin). Which of the following statements indicates that he understands the adverse effects of this medication?
   a. "If I have difficulty with balance or walking, I will contact my physician."
   b. "I will call my physician if I experience headaches."
   c. "I may have a low-grade fever late in the afternoon."
   d. "I can anticipate diarrhea, so I will avoid foods high in roughage."

7. Which of the following medications, if administered concurrently with aspirin, will increase its effects?
   a. Ascorbic acid (vitamin C)
   b. Misoprostol (Cytotec)
   c. Sodium bicarbonate
   d. Thiazide diuretics

8. Your client is started on cyclophosphamide (Cytoxan). Which of the following lab values should be assessed on a regular basis?
   a. Hematocrit
   b. WBC
   c. Uric acid levels
   d. Serum glucose

9. Mr. B. is admitted with visual changes, drowsiness, hearing difficulty, confusion, and hyperventilation. These symptoms may be attributable to
   a. acute acetaminophen (Tylenol) poisoning.
   b. salicylate intoxication.
   c. acute ergot poisoning.
   d. hyperuricemia.

10. Your client has started taking aspirin for the pain and stiffness associated with arthritis. When can he or she expect to see improvement of symptoms?
    a. 3–4 hours
    b. 6–12 hours
    c. 24–48 hours
    d. 48–72 hours

■ Critical Thinking Case Study

Mr. J., a 55-year-old teacher, has been prescribed sulindac (Clinoril) for rheumatoid arthritis that has been unresponsive to other drugs. In reviewing Mr. J.'s record, you find that he has a history of psychosis, diabetes, hypertension, and anemia.

1. Identify what in the client's history should be discussed with the physician before sulindac (Clinoril) is started and why.

2. Identify the periodic assessments that will be planned for this client.

3. Discuss the teaching you will do with this client.

Mr. J. is experiencing severe pain. His physician prescribes ketorolac (Toradol).

4. Describe how you will explain the rationale for the change in medication to the client.

CHAPTER 8

Antianxiety and Sedative-Hypnotic Drugs

■ Fill in the Blanks

1. When anxiety is _____, it impairs the ability to function.

2. The classification of anxiety disorder includes _____, _____, _____, _____, _____, and _____.

3. REM (____) sleep is thought to be _____ _____.

4. Insomnia may be caused by _____, _____, _____, _____, and _____.

5. _____, _____, and other drugs are used to treat anxiety and insomnia.

6. Four major problems associated with barbiturate use were _____, _____, _____, and _____.

7. Benzodiazepines may cause _____ and _____ dependence.

8. Benzodiazepines are _____ soluble and bind to _____.

9. Several benzodiazepines have a _____ half-life and require _____ days to reach a steady state.

10. Buspirone (_____) causes less _____ and does not cause _____ or _____ dependence but lacks the _____ and _____ effects of benzodiazepines.

11. Hydroxyzine (_____) has _____ and _____ properties.

12. _____, the oldest sedative-hypnotic, is _____, effective, and _____, but _____ develops quickly.

13. Antihistamines such as _____ (_____) also cause drowsiness.

14. Benzodiazepines are used as _____, _____, and _____ agents. They are also used for preoperative sedation and to prevent _____ and _____ in acute alcohol withdrawal.

15. Benzodiazepines are contraindicated in _____, _____ or _____, and _____ and for clients with a history of _____.

16. Clinical manifestations of benzodiazepine withdrawal syndrome include _____, _____, _____, _____, _____, _____, and _____. More serious manifestations include _____, _____, _____, _____, and _____.

17. _____ (_____) is an antidote for benzodiazepines.

18. In the presence of liver disease, the benzodiazepines of choice are _____ (_____) and _____ (_____).

■ Definitions

Define the following terms.

1. Anxiety

   _____

   _____

   _____

2. Insomnia

   _____

   _____

   _____

3. REM sleep

   _____

   _____

   _____

4. Enzyme induction

   _____

   _____

   _____

■ Nursing Diagnosis

Mrs. J., a 38-year-old woman, has recently been diagnosed with ALS (amyotrophic lateral sclerosis). She is extremely anxious and her physician has placed her on antianxiety medication. Identify three possible nursing diagnoses, pertinent assessment data, and nursing interventions.

1. Nursing Diagnosis:

   Assessment Data:

   Nursing Interventions:

2. Nursing Diagnosis:

   Assessment Data:

   Nursing Interventions:

3. Nursing Diagnosis:

   Assessment Data:

   Nursing Interventions:

■ Review Questions

1. Ms. A. has been using alprazolam (Xanax) for 1 week for insomnia. She states that she is sleeping at night but does not feel rested. This is probably due to a reduction in
   a. stage I sleep.
   b. stage II sleep.
   c. stage III sleep.
   d. REM sleep.

2. The following instruction should be given to clients who are to receive alprazolam (Xanax):
   a. "If you experience drowsiness, discontinue the medication."
   b. "Avoid alcohol."
   c. "If you are unable to sleep at night, take 1½ tablets."
   d. "Take the medication as you need it for anxiety."

3. Abruptly stopping alprazolam (Xanax) can result in
   a. seizures.
   b. headaches.
   c. dermatitis.
   d. rebound tachycardia.

4. You should assess a client receiving benzodiazepines for
   a. reduced albumin.
   b. elevated creatinine.
   c. elevated bilirubin.
   d. reduced platelets.

5. When a benzodiazepine is administered preoperatively for sleep, you should instruct the client that he or she can anticipate the desired effect within
   a. 15 minutes.
   b. 90 minutes.
   c. 45 minutes.
   d. 60 minutes.

6. A sedative that is also used as a skeletal muscle relaxant is
   a. alprazolam (Xanax).
   b. diazepam (Valium).
   c. midazolam (Versed).
   d. lorazepam (Ativan).

7. Benzodiazepines
   a. potentiate effects of other CNS depressants.
   b. produce little dependence when given as recommended.
   c. are associated with gastritis when given with caffeine.
   d. are absorbed slowly when given orally.

8. Chlordiazepoxide (Librium)
   a. peaks rapidly when administered intramuscularly.
   b. has no cumulative effects.
   c. may be used for treating alcohol withdrawal.
   d. is used for situational anxiety.

9. The benzodiazepine associated with memory impairment is
   a. alprazolam (Xanax).
   b. diazepam (Valium).
   c. midazolam (Versed).
   d. lorazepam (Ativan).

10. Antianxiety medications
    a. only need to be administered for 2 weeks.
    b. eliminate all feelings of distress.
    c. aid in symptomatic relief.
    d. produce a cure for anxiety reactions.

CHAPTER 9

Antipsychotic Drugs

■ Fill in the Blanks

Complete the following sentences.

1. _____ is a severe mental disorder characterized by disorganized and often bizarre thinking.

2. _____ are perceptions of people or objects that are not present.

3. _____ are false beliefs that persist in the absence of evidence.

4. Symptoms of _____ usually begin in adolescence or early adulthood.

5. _____ is the most common chronic psychosis.

6. Acute psychosis may be precipitated by _____, _____, and _____.

7. Phenothiazine exerts many pharmacologic effects, including _____, _____, _____, and _____.

8. Antipsychotic drugs decrease the effects of _____.

9. Manifestations of hyperarousal are _____, _____, _____, _____, or _____ behavior.

10. Clinical indications for the use of antipsychotics that are not associated with psychiatric illness include treatment of _____, _____, and intractable hiccups.

11. Promethazine (_____) is used for its _____, _____, and _____ effects.

12. Chlorprothixene (_____) and thiothixene (_____) are used for their _____ effects.

13. Haloperidol (_____) produces a _____ incidence of _____ and _____ and a _____ incidence of _____.

14. Haldol is also used in _____, _____, and _____.

15. Extrapyramidal effects produced by some antipsychotic medications include _____, _____, _____, and _____.

16. Loxapine (_____) and clozapine (_____) are used for the treatment of schizophrenia. Clozapine has a high risk of _____ and may cause other adverse effects, including _____, _____, _____, and weight gain.

17. Pimozide (Orap) is used for the treatment of _____. Serious adverse effects include _____, _____, and _____.

18. Goals of treatment with antipsychotic drugs are to _____, _____, and _____.

19. Some clients who do not respond well to one type of antipsychotic drug may require _____. This substitution must be done gradually. Abrupt substitution may cause _____.

20. Clients who are unable or unwilling to take daily doses of antipsychotic drugs may be given _____ of _____.

21. The best time to administer antipsychotic drugs is _____ daily at _____.

22. African Americans tend to respond to antipsychotics _____ and experience a higher incidence of _____ than whites.

23. Asians metabolize antipsychotic drugs _____ and have a _____ plasma drug level for a given dose than whites.

24. Anticholinergic effects include _____, _____, _____, _____, _____, and _____.

25. Clients should be taught to practice good oral hygiene, including _____, _____, _____, and _____.

■ Caution or Contraindication

*Place **ca** in front of the conditions for which antipsychotic medications should be used with **caution** and **ci** in front of the conditions for which the use of antipsychotics is **contraindicated**.*

1. _____ Liver damage
2. _____ Coronary artery disease
3. _____ CVA
4. _____ Seizure disorders
5. _____ Diabetes mellitus
6. _____ Parkinson's disease
7. _____ Glaucoma
8. _____ Peptic ulcer disease
9. _____ Bone marrow depression
10. _____ Hypertension
11. _____ Chronic respiratory disorders
12. _____ Severe depressive states
13. _____ Coma

■ Word Find

Place the trade name next to the generic name, then circle the trade name in the word find.

1. acetophenazine _____
2. thioridazine _____
3. prochlorperazine _____
4. fluphenazine hydrochloride _____
5. chlorpromazine _____
6. perphenazine _____
7. promazine _____
8. trifluoperazine _____
9. molindone _____
10. pimozide _____
11. clozapine _____
12. haloperidol _____
13. chlorprothixene _____
14. thiothixene _____
15. loxapine _____

WORD FIND

```
T A L E F D F D Q C N Q N S P A R I N E T X A T W
A N C O E K N U M O A R D I Q N B P N T P T M I H
R G P T M T M I G J F U W T C Y I I D E O M R G K
A G G L I I S T M N P K R O T E Z R E N R E Z N X
C L L W I N E F I C D E L S N A X U O W Y O Z A R
T Y O N R D G S D B P W B R P R O T V S P Q V Y L
A V G E M A A O R H P H I M E V K O F N M H T M I
N Z R B T L C L O I X M O B A N I X E U Z Y R N G
R H V T G H F J J N A C L O Z A R I L E A Z I H O
A T L Y A Z O Y B I D L E S P X T F N D N S L S V
D F H I M D F R U T P T O R T I D S H L B Z A T E
X O N A B Q S O A R P P T I U O N D C O W N F C I
R U C N K I V O V Z A S H Q O I P C P X R A O L Z
F K J K Z X C Z A M I B T A N D A O A I P V N C D
G C D T X E C F J G E N F G L X H O L T E B T M O
C D T I P B Q T U D H L E R A D P D A A P X D A T
P L A A W S M A X V T G L A A G O N P N A P E C N
O R R N I U O Q U S P U S A V A S L G E O N E I Q
P O F E J N T N A N Y L K I R S B N C L K I S N L
O K C P L V R N A I A Y J R E I C L N O S W T Y H
P E A R B S E R E V C X T S T E L A Z I N E T O S
P R O L I X I N X A A S O N I Q U G P E N T A N Y
L K I S N G L O O K L N R N A Y J R E C L I N O S
T Y H P E A M B E R E C E P X T O S H R F R N O H
H M A Z Y P X D R M B B L K A O T R I L U A A C B
```

■ Review Questions

1. Six weeks after starting chlorpromazine (Thorazine), Mrs. P. complains of difficulty chewing and swallowing. You should
   a. crush Mrs. P.'s medications.
   b. place Mrs. P. on a full liquid diet.
   c. puree all Mrs. P.'s food.
   d. contact the physician.

2. Your client is taking chlorpromazine (Thorazine). The following symptom should be reported to the physician immediately.
   a. Loss of appetite
   b. Dry mouth
   c. Diarrhea
   d. Sore throat

3. Mrs. T.'s husband is dying of cancer, and he is psychotic and extremely agitated. His physician orders haloperidol (Haldol) 2 mg q2h PRN until his symptoms are controlled. Mrs. T. asks you when Mr. T.'s symptoms will be controlled. Your best response would be the following:
   a. "It will take three or four doses before we see any results."
   b. "He should begin to calm down within the hour."
   c. "The symptoms are usually controlled within 72 hours."
   d. "If we medicate him every 2 hours around the clock, he will be calm by tomorrow morning."

4. Your client is presently taking propranolol (Inderal). Her physician starts her on perphenazine (Trilafon) for psychosis. You know that
   a. the dosage of Trilafon may need to be increased because she is using Inderal.
   b. the dosage of Trilafon may need to be decreased because she is using Inderal.
   c. the dosage of Inderal may need to be increased because Trilafon was added.
   d. no change in dosage needs to be made.

5. M.J. is admitted for a psychotic episode. He attempts to bite an orderly while he is being restrained. When you administer IM chlorpromazine (Thorazine) to M.J., you should

   a. question him about his feelings.

   b. demonstrate a calm, firm manner.

   c. ask him where he would like the injection.

   d. wait for him to calm down.

6. Which of these statements by your client, who has been started on perphenazine (Trilafon), indicates that she understands the instructions you have given her?

   a. "I will see my dentist every six months and brush my teeth frequently."

   b. "I will only go outside at night."

   c. "I will lie down for an hour after each dose of the medication."

   d. "I will take antacids with my medication."

7. When doing discharge teaching with your client who is taking thioridazine (Mellaril), which of the following instructions is appropriate?

   a. "You need to see the doctor weekly to have a white blood cell count done."

   b. "Use a sunscreen and wear protective clothing when out in the sun."

   c. "A diet high in fiber with a good fluid intake will help you maintain normal bowel habits."

   d. "Discontinue the medication if you are drowsy or dizzy."

8. Mr. H., who is taking antipsychotic medication, starts smacking his lips, protruding his tongue, and engaging in facial grimacing. Based on these findings, the nurse should suspect

   a. increased psychosis.

   b. dystonia.

   c. tardive dyskinesia.

   d. Parkinsonism.

9. After assessing Mrs. J., who has just been admitted to your unit, you obtain the following data: BP 160/70, pulse 98, respiration 26, temperature 96.2°F. Which one of these findings could be attributed to the use of antipsychotic medications?

   a. Blood pressure

   b. Pulse

   c. Respiration

   d. Temperature

10. The best time to administer oral antipsychotic drugs that are ordered once a day is

   a. upon awakening.

   b. with breakfast.

   c. before dinner.

   d. 1–2 hours before bedtime.

■ Critical Thinking Case Study

Mr. P., an 89-year-old, is admitted from home with a diagnosis of psychosis. He is agitated and combative. The following laboratory tests were ordered: SGOT/AST, WBC, Na^+, K^+, Cl^-, glucose.

1. Identify medical conditions in which the use of antipsychotic medications would be contraindicated.

Mr. J. is started on fluphenazine hydrochloride (Prolixin) IM.

2. Determine what an appropriate dose for Mr. P. would be and discuss how you came to the conclusion.

3. Discuss why this medication was chosen.

Mr. P.'s daughter is very concerned about him and asks when she can expect to see improvement in his condition.

4. Discuss your response to Mr. P.'s daughter.

Four days after admission, Mr. P.'s daughter is very upset because he is sleeping all the time.

5. Explain to Mr. P.'s daughter what she can expect.

One month after admission, Mr. P. develops compulsive, involuntary, restless movements. Mr. P.'s daughter questions whether the psychosis has returned.

6. Describe your response to Mr. P.'s daughter.

Mr. P.'s daughter plans on taking him home to live with her.

7. Discuss what instructions she should be given.

Copyright © 2001. Lippincott Williams & Wilkins.
Study Guide to Accompany Clinical Drug Therapy: Rationales for Nursing Practice, sixth edition, by Gail Ropelewski-Ryan.

CHAPTER 10

Antidepressants

■ Fill in the Blanks

Complete the following sentences.

1. Symptoms of depression include

   a. _____

   b. _____

   c. _____

   d. _____

   e. _____

   f. _____

   g. _____

   h. _____

   i. _____

   j. _____

   k. _____

2. Secondary depression may be precipitated by _____, _____, _____, and _____.

3. Tricyclic antidepressants (TCAs) produce _____, _____, and cardiac dysrhythmias.

4. Amitriptyline (_____) is a commonly used _____.

5. Fluoxetine (_____), a selective serotonin reuptake inhibitor (SSRI), can produce common adverse effects, including _____, _____, _____, and _____.

6. When Prozac is discontinued, it can take _____ for the drug to be eliminated from the body.

7. Monoamine oxidase (MAO) inhibitors may interact with _____ and _____ to produce _____.

8. Foods that interact with MAO inhibitors are those containing _____.

9. List eight commonly eaten foods that are high in tyramine.

   a. _____

   b. _____

   c. _____

   d. _____

   e. _____

   f. _____

   g. _____

   h. _____

10. Lithium carbonate (_____) is used for clients with _____.

11. _____ is a prerequisite for lithium therapy.

12. Deviations in serum _____ affect lithium levels.

13. A therapeutic effect from lithium is expected in _____ days.

14. TCAs are used in children and adolescents for _____.

15. SSRIs may be used for _____.

16. It takes _____ weeks before the therapeutic effects from MAOs are seen.

17. Symptoms associated with a SSRI overdose include: _____, _____, _____, _____, and _____.

18. Adverse effects seen with toxic drug levels (above 2.5 mEq/L) of lithium include _____, _____, _____, _____, and _____, _____, _____, _____, _____ and _____.

▪ Sentence Correction

Circle the word that makes the sentence incorrect and place the correct word in the space provided. Example:
contraindicated *Antidepressants are* (commonly used) *for clients with schizophrenia.*

1. _____ An adverse effect of antidepressants that is useful in treating enuresis is insomnia.

2. _____ Furosemide (Lasix) should not be administered with MAO inhibitors because a hypertensive crisis could occur.

3. _____ A deficiency of potassium increases the risk of lithium toxicity.

4. _____ Fluoxetine (Prozac) needs to be administered b.i.d.

5. _____ Blurred vision should be reported to the physician for persons taking MAO inhibitors.

6. _____ Adequate hepatic function is a prerequisite for lithium therapy.

7. _____ Depression results from a deficiency of dopamine and norepinephrine.

8. _____ Tricyclic antidepressants produce a relatively high incidence of cardiac failure.

9. _____ Gastric lavage is the preferred treatment for lithium overdose.

10. _____ TCAs are the drug of choice for older adults.

11. _____ If therapeutic effects from TCAs are not seen in 8 weeks, the medication should be discontinued.

12. _____ Lithium is used to control severe depression.

13. _____ Most antidepressants cause hypertension.

14. _____ Serum lithium levels should be drawn every 6 months.

15. _____ TCAs are not recommended for persons under the age of 18 except for treatment of enuresis; then they may be used in children over age 12.

▪ Critical Thinking Case Study

Mrs. J., a 48-year-old homemaker whose daughter entered college this fall, is admitted to your unit with a diagnosis of depression.

1. Discuss how the diagnosis of depression is made.

Mrs. J. has a history of diabetes, gout, COPD, and allergies to pollen and animal dander.

2. Identify which of Mrs. J.'s illnesses need to be considered before antidepressants are prescribed.

The physician starts Mrs. J. on fluoxetine (Prozac).

3. Identify appropriate goals for Mrs. J.

4. Specify the instruction Mrs. J. should be given before going home.

Mrs. J. returns to the clinic 3 weeks after starting antidepressant therapy complaining of anxiety and insomnia. Mrs. J. states that she is feeling worse and does not want to continue the medication.

5. Identify the assessments you will do.

6. Discuss how you will deal with Mrs. J.'s unwillingness to continue the medication.

■ Review Questions

1. Which of the following nursing actions take priority when caring for Mr. J., who is taking lithium?
   a. Monitor peripheral pulses.
   b. Provide a diet high in potassium.
   c. Provide a stimulating environment.
   d. Monitor fluid and electrolyte intake.

2. Foods that should be eliminated from the diet when a person is taking MAO inhibitors include
   a. oranges.
   b. chicken.
   c. eggs.
   d. cheese.

3. A client is admitted with a diagnosis of overdose of bupropion (Wellbutrin). Which of the following nursing diagnoses would be a priority?
   a. Potential for injury related to seizure activity.
   b. Knowledge deficit related to effects and usage of antidepressant.
   c. Sleep pattern disturbances related to depression.
   d. Alteration in thought process related to confusion.

4. Mr. J., diagnosed with bipolar affective disorder, is to be started on lithium. He is taking aspirin, digoxin (Lanoxin), insulin, and furosemide (Lasix). Which of these medications must you make the physician aware of before you start the lithium?
   a. Aspirin
   b. Digoxin (Lanoxin)
   c. Insulin
   d. Furosemide (Lasix)

5. Which of the following medications, if administered concurrently with MAO inhibitors, will increase their effect?
   a. Hydrochlorothiazide (Oretic)
   b. Sodium bicarbonate
   c. Theophylline
   d. Meperidine (Demerol)

6. The nurse should assess the client who is taking lithium for symptoms of toxicity, which include
   a. bradycardia, hypotension, and apnea.
   b. blurred vision and polydipsia.
   c. fever and rash of the head and neck.
   d. tremors, oliguria, and confusion.

7. Which of the following statements by the client leads you to believe that he has understood the teaching that you have done regarding tricyclic antidepressants?
   a. "It is common to experience diarrhea. I will increase the fiber in my diet."
   b. "I may feel drowsy for a few weeks after the medication is started."
   c. "Nausea and vomiting are common in the first few weeks. I will eat small, frequent meals."
   d. "Skin rashes are common occurrences. I will stay out of the sun."

8. A lithium level is drawn, and it is 2.6 mEq/L. You know that this level is
   a. below the therapeutic range.
   b. within the therapeutic range.
   c. slightly above the therapeutic range.
   d. indicative of severe toxicity.

9. When phenelzine (Nardil) is initiated, the nurse should assess the client for
   a. ataxia.
   b. hypotension.
   c. diarrhea.
   d. hyperglycemia.

10. A client who started taking lithium 2 days ago developed hand tremors. The best nursing action in this instance would be to
   a. administer propranolol (Inderal) to control the tremors.
   b. hold the lithium until the tremors subside.
   c. assure him that this is common and usually subsides within a few weeks.
   d. contact the physician immediately; stay with the client and have him remain in bed.

CHAPTER 11

Antiseizure Drugs

■ Fill in the Blanks

Complete the following sentences.

1. A seizure is a _____.
   _____.

2. A convulsion is a _____.
   _____.

3. Epilepsy is a _____.
   _____.

4. Epilepsy is diagnosed with an _____.

5. When epilepsy begins in infancy, causes include
   _____, _____, or
   _____.

6. Status epilepticus can be induced as a result of
   overdose of the following drugs:
   _____, _____,
   _____.

7. Common adverse effects of phenytoin (Dilantin)
   include: _____,
   _____, _____,
   _____, _____, and
   _____.

8. _____ (Tegretol) is used for clients
   with _____, _____, and
   _____ seizures. It is also used to
   treat facial pain associated with _____.

9. Diazepam (_____) and lorazepam
   (_____) are used to terminate
   _____.

10. The following may produce seizures in people with
    no previous history of seizures: _____,
    _____, hypoxia, hypoglycemia,
    _____, and withdrawal from CNS
    depressants.

11. For most clients, anticonvulsant therapy is
    _____.

12. Discontinuing or changing antiseizure drugs must
    be done over _____ or
    _____.

13. Phenytoin (Dilantin), given intravenously, can
    _____. It should not be given to
    clients with _____ or
    _____.

14. _____ is the anticonvulsant of
    choice for status epilepticus.

15. Many anticonvulsants decrease levels of
    _____, which can lead to mega-
    loblastic anemia.

■ True or False

1. _____ A toxic level of lidocaine can produce
   seizures.

2. _____ During a seizure, a spoon should be inserted between the teeth to protect the tongue.

3. _____ Tonic-clonic seizures can result in agnosia,
   which lasts 3–4 hours after the seizure is
   over.

4. _____ Most anticonvulsant drugs have the potential for causing blood, liver, and kidney
   disorders.

5. _____ Oral anticonvulsants should be administered on an empty stomach.

6. _____ Alcohol increases the effect of phenytoin
   (Dilantin).

7. _____ Weight gain is common with persons taking anticonvulsant drugs.

■ Crossword Puzzle

ACROSS

2. A tolerance to this drug can occur with long-term use.
4. A benzodiazepine used for acute alcohol withdrawal and to manage partial seizures.
5. The drug of choice for treating status epilepticus.
9. An anticonvulsant that is often used in conjunction with Dilantin.

DOWN

1. A type of seizure characterized by spasmodic reactions.
3. May cause life-threatening blood dyscrasia.
6. The initial drug of choice in adults who are experiencing tonic-clonic seizures.
7. Used to treat absence and mixed seizures.
8. A brain disorder that causes seizures.
10. Used to terminate acute seizures.

■ Review Questions

1. The most important nursing diagnosis for a newly admitted client with a seizure disorder is
   a. risk for injury.
   b. ineffective coping.
   c. knowledge deficit.
   d. self-care deficit.

2. The drug of choice for treating generalized seizures in infants is
   a. phenobarbital.
   b. clonazepam (Klonopin).
   c. phenytoin (Dilantin).
   d. diazepam (Valium).

3. A therapeutic phenobarbital level is
   a. 2–7 µg/mL.
   b. 10–25 µg/mL.
   c. 25–50 µg/mL.
   d. 40–50 µg/mL.

4. Which of the following drugs is most effective for treating acute alcohol withdrawal?
   a. Carbamazepine (Tegretol)
   b. Clonazepam (Klonopin)
   c. Clorazepate (Tranxene)
   d. Ethosuximide (Zarontin)

5. The dosage of phenytoin (Dilantin) may need to be adjusted if your client is taking
   a. beta blockers.
   b. anticholinergics.
   c. oral contraceptives.
   d. calcium channel blockers.

6. Persons taking valproic acid (Depakene) must be observed for
   a. abnormal liver function.
   b. weight gain.
   c. night blindness.
   d. abnormal blood glucose levels.

7. Mr. J. is in ICU after open heart surgery. He is receiving theophylline, digoxin, Nipride, and nitroglycerin. Mr. J. experiences a seizure. A toxic effect from which of the drugs that he is receiving could have produced the seizure?

   a. Theophylline

   b. Nipride

   c. Digoxin

   d. Nitroglycerin

8. Ms. M. is admitted to the ER and begins to have rapid rhythmic and symmetric jerking movements of her body. You would document this as a

   a. partial seizure.

   b. focal seizure.

   c. petit mal seizure.

   d. major motor seizure.

9. When administering a loading dose of phenytoin (Dilantin), the nurse should observe the client closely for

   a. hypertension.

   b. respiratory depression.

   c. hypotension.

   d. decreased level of consciousness.

10. Your client is receiving 100 mg of phenytoin (Dilantin) b.i.d. His Dilantin level is 30 µg/mL. You would expect to

   a. administer the dosage as ordered.

   b. decrease the daily dosage.

   c. hold the drug until further orders.

   d. increase the daily dosage.

■ Critical Thinking Case Study

C.M., a 16-year-old female, was admitted to your unit with a head injury following an automobile accident. She has been having intermittent seizures since her hospitalization 24 hours ago. (Learners may need to use additional sources to answer these questions.)

1. Describe what you will do if C.M. has another seizure.

The physician initially prescribed phenytoin (Dilantin) 100 mg b.i.d. and phenobarbital 20 mg b.i.d. for C.M.

2. Discuss why her physician ordered two anticonvulsants.

After 2 days, C.M. develops a rash all over her body.

3. Identify your nursing actions in response to C.M.'s rash.

C.M. asks you if she will have to take the medication the rest of her life.

4. Describe your response.

C.M. is discharged on primidone (Mysoline).

5. Describe the teaching that you will do before discharge.

CHAPTER 12

Antiparkinson Drugs

■ Fill in the Blanks

Complete the following sentences.

1. Parkinson's disease is a _____, _____, _____ disorder of the CNS characterized by abnormalities in movement and posture, _____, _____, and _____.

2. Classic parkinsonism results from destruction of _____.

3. Dopaminergic drugs that exert beneficial effects in Parkinson's disease are:
   levadopa (_____)
   carbidopa (_____)
   amantadine (_____)
   bromocriptine (_____)
   pergolide (_____)
   pramipexole (_____)
   ropinirole (_____)
   selegiline (_____)
   and tolcapone (_____).

4. Amantadine (_____) increases _____.

5. Bromocriptine (Parlodel) stimulates _____.

6. Selegiline blocks the enzyme _____, which _____ dopamine.

7. Tolcapone blocks the enzyme _____.

8. Levodopa (Larodopa, Dopar) is the _____ drug available for the treatment of Parkinson's disease.

9. With long-term use of levodopa (Dopar), clients experience _____ of parkinsonism symptoms.

10. A levodopa-carbidopa combination product is _____, which allows more levodopa to reach the _____.

11. Amantadine (_____) relieves parkinsonism symptoms in _____ days, but loses its effectiveness in 6–8 weeks of continuous administration.

12. Bromocriptine (Parlodel) stimulates _____.

13. Pramipexole (_____) and ropinirole (_____) are approved for _____ and _____ stages of Parkinson's disease.

■ True or False

1. _____ Levodopa (Dopar) and bromocriptine (Parlodel) should be given on an empty stomach.

2. _____ Anticholinergic drugs produce atropine-like effects.

3. _____ Dyskinesia is a side effect of levodopa and results in involuntary movements of the tongue, mouth, face, or whole body.

4. _____ Persons taking levodopa should be observed for bradycardia.

5. _____ Bromocriptine (Parlodel) can produce a patchy blue discoloration of the skin on the legs, called livedo reticularis.

6. _____ Persons taking levodopa need to increase their intake of protein and vitamin B_6.

7. _____ Selegiline (Eldepryl) can cause hypertension if the client ingests foods containing tyramine.

■ Review Questions

1. Your client is to go home on levodopa (Dopar). Which of the following statements leads you to believe that he has understood the teaching you have done?
   a. "I will limit my fluid intake to 1500 mL a day."
   b. "I will avoid yellow vegetables."
   c. "I will increase the fiber in my diet."
   d. "I will limit my intake of alcohol and protein."

2. Levodopa is contraindicated for use in persons who have
   a. migraine headaches.
   b. peptic ulcer disease.
   c. thyroid disease.
   d. glaucoma.

3. Amantadine hydrochloride (Symmetrel) can produce
   a. constipation.
   b. mottling and swelling of the extremities.
   c. dyskinesia.
   d. sluggish pupillary response.

4. Which of the following is an adverse effect from levodopa that commonly occurs in the first few weeks of therapy?
   a. Hallucinations
   b. Diarrhea
   c. Hypotension
   d. Urinary retention

5. The physician plans to start your client on trihexyphenidyl (Artane). Which of the following assessments would warrant holding the medication until the physician had been contacted?
   a. Pulse of 102
   b. BP of 88/60
   c. Temperature of 100.2°F
   d. Respirations 14

6. You should assess Mrs. C., who is receiving Sinemet (levodopa-carbidopa), for the following adverse reaction:
   a. paralytic ileus.
   b. gastrointestinal bleeding.
   c. cardiac dysrhythmias.
   d. hypotension.

7. Mr. P., age 75, is taking anticholinergic agents for Parkinson's disease and as a result is experiencing decreased sweating. This places him at a risk for experiencing
   a. dehydration.
   b. fluid volume overload.
   c. dry skin.
   d. heat stroke.

8. The following medication is an MAO inhibitor used for the treatment of Parkinson's disease:
   a. amantadine (Symmetrel)
   b. selegiline (Eldepryl)
   c. ropinirole (Requip)
   d. pramipexole (Mirapex).

9. Before administering selegiline (Eldepryl), you should ask your client if he has a history of
   a. diabetes mellitus.
   b. hypertension.
   c. peripheral vascular disease.
   d. pulmonary disease.

10. Tolcapone (Tasmar) is a new type of antiparkinsonian drugs called a(an)
    a. anticholinergic agent.
    b. MAO inhibitor.
    c. catecholomethyltransferase inhibitor.
    d. dopamine antagonist.

■ Critical Thinking Case Study

Mr. P. is diagnosed with Parkinson's disease and started on benztropine (Cogentin), an anticholinergic agent.

1. Identify why Mr. P. was started on Cogentin.

2. Identify the adverse effects of this medication and the nursing measures that you will employ to prevent complications.

5. Identify what you will assess Mr. P. for, and what you will teach the client.

Mr. P. asks you about the progression of Parkinson's disease.

3. Describe how you will respond to his inquiry.

6. Identify your instructions prior to discharge.

Two years after initial diagnosis, the medication Mr. P. is receiving is no longer effective and the physician starts Mr. P. on pramipexole (Mirapex).

4. Discuss why this medication was chosen for Mr. P.

CHAPTER 13

Skeletal Muscle Relaxants

■ Fill in the Blanks

Complete the following sentences.

1. Skeletal muscle relaxants are used to
_____ or _____.

2. _____ is the only muscle relaxant
that acts on the muscle itself.

3. Dantrolene (Dantrium) is also indicated for prevention and treatment of _____.

4. For acute muscle relaxation, drugs that can be
given IV include _____
(_____) and _____
(_____).

5. The drug of choice for persons with multiple sclerosis is _____.

6. Adjunctive measures for muscle spasm include
   a. _____.
   b. _____.
   c. _____.
   d. _____.

7. Muscle relaxants have not been established as safe
for use in _____.

8. While taking muscle relaxants, clients should be
instructed to avoid activities that require
_____ or _____.

9. Skeletal muscle relaxants should be administered
with _____. This minimizes the risk
of _____.

10. If baclofen (_____) is stopped
abruptly, it can cause _____.

■ True or False

1. _____ Dantrolene (Dantrium) is used for the
treatment of malignant hyperthermia.

2. _____ If hypersensitivity reactions occur, the
dosage of the drug should be decreased.

3. _____ Persons taking MAO inhibitors will need
to increase their dose of muscle relaxants
to produce the same effect.

4. _____ Diazepam (Valium) can produce psychological or physical dependence.

5. _____ The dosage of muscle relaxants should be
increased slowly.

6. _____ Rapid IV administration of skeletal muscle
relaxants can result in hypertension.

■ Crossword Puzzle

ACROSS

2. An adverse effect of skeletal muscle relaxants.

3. Approved for treating people with multiple sclerosis.

4. A muscle relaxant that should be administered with food to prevent GI distress.

6. Persons with a spinal cord injury can experience _____.

8. The drug for prevention and treatment of malignant hyperthermia.

9. Skeletal muscle relaxants have not been proven safe for use during _____.

10. The patient should lie down while this drug is being administered via IV.

DOWN

1. A nonpharmacological intervention for muscle spasm.

5. Be cautious using this drug in persons with glaucoma or dysrhythmias.

7. Physically incompatible with other drugs of this class.

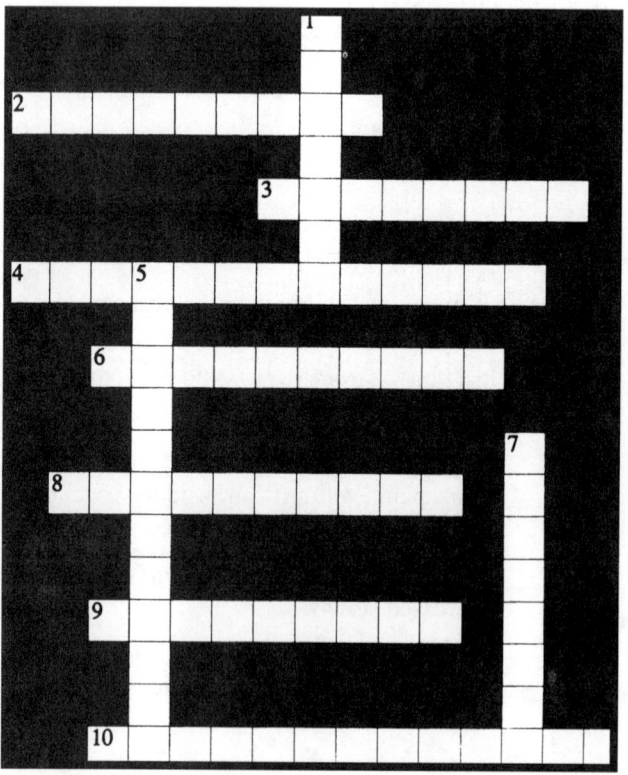

■ Review Questions

1. The following muscle relaxant is also used to treat malignant hyperthermia:
   a. dantrolene (Dantrium).
   b. diazepam (Valium).
   c. baclofen (Lioresal).
   d. carisoprodol (Soma).

2. The muscle relaxant of choice for clients who are pregnant is
   a. methocarbamol (Robaxin).
   b. diazepam (Valium).
   c. baclofen (Lioresal).
   d. none of the above.

3. A muscle relaxant that can be administered parenterally for acute muscle spasm is
   a. metaxalone (Skelaxin).
   b. baclofen (Lioresal).
   c. cyclobenzaprine (Flexeril).
   d. methocarbamol (Robaxin).

4. Which of the following statements indicates that your client, who is receiving dantrolene (Dantrium), has understood the teaching that you have done?
   a. "I will not stop my medication if I experience side effects. I will contact my physician."
   b. "I will limit my alcohol and caffeine intake while I am taking this medication."
   c. "The medicine may cause decreased tolerance to cold."
   d. "The medicine will prevent the progression of my multiple sclerosis."

5. Mr. H. is started on dantrolene (Dantrium) for muscle spasticity. Which of the following laboratory studies should be monitored when the medication is administered?
   a. Hematocrit and hemoglobin
   b. SGOT and LDH
   c. CPK (MB)
   d. Creatinine clearance

6. The maximum recommended length of treatment with metaxalone (Skelaxin) is
   a. 2–3 consecutive days.
   b. 10 consecutive days.
   c. 2 consecutive weeks.
   d. 4 consecutive weeks.

7. The following group of medications, if administered concurrently with muscle relaxants, will increase the risk of respiratory depression:

   a. antihistamines.

   b. antihypertensives.

   c. antidiabetic agents.

   d. antiseizure agents.

8. When teaching Mrs. S. about the effects of baclofen (Lioresal), you should include the following information:

   a. "The medication should be taken with milk or meals."

   b. "You should expect a drop in your pulse rate."

   c. "If you experience drowsiness, contact your physician immediately."

   d. "Skin rashes are expected and will go away in a few weeks."

9. The following group using dantrolene (Dantrium) is at greater risk for developing hepatotoxicity:

   a. insulin-dependent clients with diabetes.

   b. hypertensive clients with renal impairment.

   c. men over 55 with prostate disease.

   d. women over 35 taking estrogen.

10. The following is an expected outcome when methocarbamol (Robaxin) is administered for acute muscle spasms:

    a. increased tolerance to heat and cold.

    b. increased physical coordination.

    c. increased ability to maintain posture and balance.

    d. increased mobility and decreased pain.

■ Critical Thinking Case Study

Joe Smith, a high school senior, injured his ankle in a football game. His physician ordered metaxalone (Skelaxin) to relieve the pain associated with an ankle injury. Two weeks after his initial injury, he returned to his physician's office still complaining of pain and requesting a prescription renewal.

1. Identify the assessments that you will do.

2. Describe your response to his request for additional medication.

3. Discuss alternatives to drug therapy.

CHAPTER **14**

Anesthetics

■ Matching Exercise

TERMS AND CONCEPTS

Match the concept with the term for it.

1. _____ Decreases risk of bronchospasm.

2. _____ Added to local anesthetics to prolong their effect.

3. _____ Given intravenously to induce anesthesia.

4. _____ Given to decrease anxiety.

5. _____ Used as an antidote to reverse muscle paralysis.

6. _____ Neuromuscular blocking agent with a short duration of action.

7. _____ Adjunct to general anesthesia; to facilitate intubation.

8. _____ Used alone for analgesia in dentistry, obstetrics, and brief surgical procedures.

9. _____ A very potent opioid analgesic similar to morphine but with shorter duration.

10. _____ A naturally occurring plant alkaloid that causes skeletal muscle paralysis.

11. _____ An anticholinergic drug given to prevent vagal effects associated with surgery.

12. _____ Administration of this drug preoperatively allows easier induction of anesthesia.

13. _____ Used for short-term sedation of persons being mechanically ventilated.

14. _____ Used as a topical anesthetic for ear, nose, or throat.

15. _____ Topical anesthetic that has a rapid onset.

A. Epinephrine

B. Halothane (Fluothane)

C. Midazolam (Versed)

D. Fentanyl citrate (Sublimaze)

E. Thiopental sodium (Pentothal)

F. Tubocurarine

G. Nitrous oxide

H. Vecuronium (Norcuron)

I. Neostigmine (Prostigmin)

J. Cyclopropane

K. Succinylcholine (Anectine)

L. Glycopyrrolate (Robinul)

M. Hydroxyzine (Vistaril)

N. Propofol (Diprivan)

O. Cocaine

P. Lidocaine (Xylocaine)

■ Word Scramble

Unscramble the trade name and circle it in the word find.

1. (Enflurane) ranthee _____

2. (Isoflurane) nafoer _____

3. (Alfentanil) neatfal _____

4. (Fentanyl and droperidol) ravionn _____

5. (Pancuronium) vonpaul _____

6. (Succinylcholine) niceante _____

7. (Metocurine) neetbium _____

8. (Sufentanil) fasentu _____

9. (Midazolam) served _____

10. (Methohexital sodium) verbilat _____

■ Review Questions

1. Mr. J. was agitated and "fighting" the ventilator, so his physician ordered a medication to help maintain Mr. J. on the ventilator. Which of the following drugs will be effective for this purpose?

   a. Tetracaine (Pontocaine)

   b. Propofol (Diprivan)

   c. Thiopental sodium (Pentothal)

   d. Isoflurane (Forane)

2. Which of the following is a complication after general anesthesia that the nurse should assess for?

   a. Hypertension

   b. Bradycardia

   c. Urinary retention

   d. Hypoxia

WORD FIND

```
B A E C C T R I S O M E T A L C H E M P N I P A N
A L T B A C I T R E M E N A R C H O R O L A C O L
C M H T R A L C O H V P E R A G A R I R I H O K C
F O R A N E R L L S S N E S S T I T H E O P H Y L
T S A N S E I O E A A A N I N N O V A R E A N I X
O C N E T I P N E L A T I E N T G E O M T R I C U
B A E A L N P A L P I T F T I O N S E C O E S N E
A N E B O N D I H E X L L G H A L A B F I N I A X
C N U C T E C H Y P A V U L O N V E R E F L E X E
K A P T A B R A P P R E M E N E I O N T A O V A N
H A H S O M T R E M O R A N G C N E J T A O C N I
A B O T P E P I R N N Q B B A T T R I P C O C T N
N C R V Q T I H T E A B I E F I A R E S T L Y H H
E N I M O R B O E H T C N X O N T S E N I M A I C
C I A N S A N T N T A I N T M E T U B I N E M N Y
T A Y N A Z I T S L A E M O R D N F S S E T T E R
O M A H V O T R A C O M M R E X N E O E I F I N T
P P T A M L R T O P A M I N E C T N L B G N O I S
A H A A D O I C N A A F N N F D D T O E V E S O I
N A T I N V E R S E D I F A E L A A M M P A L O C
T I R E E E S T L E S S N E S S U A A W I T O O M
R R F R C S E T R E O N P I I A U N U T W R I M C
Y B B L R S H N V R R S I S E N I K R E P Y H C A
X T E L B E J Q U T H Y P O A C E B R S H I S P W
A L B E L L A D O W D Y M N T E S O O T Y P A K T
```

Study Guide to Accompany Clinical Drug Therapy: Rationales for Nursing Practice, sixth edition, by Gail Ropelewski-Ryan.

3. An adverse effect of isoflurane (Forane) that the nurse needs to assess for is
   a. immobility.
   b. headache.
   c. blurred vision.
   d. depressed mental alertness.

4. A common side effect, immediately after delivery, in babies whose mothers have received a local anesthetic is
   a. depressed muscle tone.
   b. cyanosis.
   c. absent bowel sounds.
   d. inability to suck.

5. Before surgery, the anesthesiologist should be made aware of any medications that will decrease the effect of the general anesthetic agents. These medications include
   a. anticholinergic medications.
   b. bronchodilators.
   c. diuretics.
   d. antihypertensive medications.

6. The anesthesiologist plans on using methoxyflurane (Penthrane) for a C-section delivery. Because of the potential toxicity from this medication, you will assess which of the following laboratory values?
   a. Chloride
   b. Blood sugar
   c. Creatinine
   d. Sodium

7. Nitrous oxide is an anesthetic that has which of the following properties?
   a. Long recovery period
   b. Many side effects
   c. Short induction period
   d. Explosive gas

8. Stage II of general anesthesia is characterized by
   a. analgesia.
   b. medullary paralysis.
   c. surgical anesthesia.
   d. excitement and hyperactivity.

9. Before administering glycopyrrolate (Robinul) preoperatively, the nurse should ask the client if he or she has a history of the following condition:
   a. glaucoma.
   b. bradycardia.
   c. hypertension.
   d. diabetes mellitus.

10. As a result of the administration of general anesthetics, postoperative patients
   a. may have difficulty voiding and will have decreased gastric motility.
   b. need to be catheterized if they have not voided within 4 hours after surgery.
   c. need large amounts of oral fluids to flush the medication out of their system.
   d. should remain on bed rest to relieve abdominal pain and distention.

■ Critical Thinking Case Study

Mrs. J., a 29-year-old woman, is admitted for a C-section. Spinal anesthesia is performed.

1. Identify two other situations in which this type of anesthesia is the preferred method.

Prior to surgery, Mrs. J. asks you what she will be able to feel during surgery.

2. Your response:

After delivery, Mrs. J. asks when she will be able to walk to the bathroom.

3. The best response would be:

4. Specify fetal responses to anesthetics that the nurse should be assessing for.

CHAPTER 15

Substance Abuse Disorders

■ Matching Exercise

TERMS AND CONCEPTS

Match the concept with the term for it.

1. _____ The primary drug of abuse worldwide.

2. _____ Symptoms of alcohol withdrawal.

3. _____ Symptoms of amphetamine withdrawal.

4. _____ Symptoms of barbiturate withdrawal.

5. _____ The use of this drug causes euphoria, increased energy, sexual arousal, tachycardia, and hypertension.

6. _____ A major danger with these drugs is their ability to impair judgment.

7. _____ These substances are most often abused by preadolescents.

8. _____ A potent analgesic that produces rapid, intense euphoria.

9. _____ This drug is used as an antiemetic for clients receiving anticancer drugs.

10. _____ A drug used in the treatment of alcohol abuse.

11. _____ A drug used in the treatment of heroin addiction.

12. _____ Symptoms seen with an overdose of opiate.

13. _____ Drug administered to reverse effects of an opiate.

14. _____ Drugs of choice for treating alcohol withdrawal.

15. _____ Treatment of an overdose of amphetamines includes these actions.

16. _____ Drug used to reverse sedation, coma, and respiratory depression caused by a benzodiazepine overdose.

A. Cocaine

B. Alcohol

C. Tremors, sweating, nausea, tachycardia

D. Heroin

E. Depression and exhaustion

F. Hallucinogenic drugs

G. Anxiety, tremors, insomnia, weight loss

H. Marijuana

I. Volatile solvents (inhalants)

J. Disulfiram (Antabuse)

K. Methadone (Dolophine)

L. Naloxone (Narcan)

M. Severe respiratory depression and coma

N. Sedation, lowering of body temperature, administration of antipsychotic drugs

O. Benzodiazepines

P. Flumazenil (Romazicon)

■ Nursing Diagnosis

Mr. Q., age 29, is admitted in hepatic coma. Identify four nursing diagnoses, assessment data, and nursing interventions for a person requiring drug treatment for alcoholism.

1. Nursing Diagnosis:

   Assessment Data:

   Nursing Interventions:

2. Nursing Diagnosis:

   Assessment Data:

   Nursing Interventions:

3. Nursing Diagnosis:

   Assessment Data:

   Nursing Interventions:

4. Nursing Diagnosis:

   Assessment Data:

   Nursing Interventions:

■ Definitions

Define the following terms.

1. Alcoholism _____

   _____

2. Psychological dependence_____

   _____

3. Physical dependence _____

   _____

■ Review Questions

1. Clients using opiates on a long-term basis are likely to become tolerant to all of the following effects except:
   a. miosis.
   b. respiratory depression.
   c. analgesia.
   d. sedation.

2. Mr. J. comes to the emergency room with a cocaine overdose. You should assess him for
   a. dysrhythmias.
   b. dyspnea.
   c. hypotension.
   d. aphasia.

3. An individual addicted to opioids would not show withdrawal symptoms if given
   a. Narcan.
   b. Stadol.
   c. Dilaudid.
   d. Nubain.

4. The following statement by Mr. C., a chronic alcoholic started on disulfiram (Antabuse), leads you to believe that he has understood your instructions. "If I drink alcohol,
   a. "it may cause my blood pressure to go up."
   b. "I must increase the amount of medication I am taking."
   c. "it may cause my blood pressure to drop."
   d. "I must decrease the amount of medication I am taking."

5. This drug is used as an antiemetic for persons receiving anticancer drugs.

   a. Cocaine

   b. Marijuana

   c. Heroin

   d. PCP

6. While Mr. G. is withdrawing from alcohol, you will

   a. encourage oral fluids to maintain hydration.

   b. withhold all medications.

   c. provide a nonstimulating environment.

   d. engage him in conversation to decrease his anxiety.

7. Mr. J. is admitted to the hospital following a car accident. He denies alcohol use, but the lab slip shows an alcohol level above the legal limit. The best approach to take is to

   a. wait until Mr. J. is ready to discuss his drinking problem.

   b. discuss the lab findings with Mr. J. and his family.

   c. confront Mr. J. with his alcohol abuse and persuade him to change.

   d. have a counselor come and see Mr. J.

8. Your client is admitted with acute amphetamine intoxication. You will observe her for

   a. somnolence and lethargy.

   b. bradycardia.

   c. hypothermia.

   d. hyperactivity and agitation.

9. Persons abusing opioids may experience

   a. acne.

   b. bruising.

   c. constipation.

   d. diarrhea.

10. J.B. is admitted with intoxication from an unknown substance. He is hyperactive, tachycardic, febrile, and hallucinating. The symptoms probably relate to an overdose of

    a. amphetamines.

    b. barbiturates.

    c. alcohol.

    d. opiates.

■ Critical Thinking Case Study

M., a 28-year-old woman, is admitted to your unit with symptoms of alcohol withdrawal. She was found on a park bench by the police. As a result of the admission blood work, you discover that M. is pregnant. (The learner may need additional resources to answer these questions.)

1. Describe how you will proceed with the admission history and physical of M.

2. Discuss how M.'s alcohol intake affects her pregnancy.

M. is anxious, agitated, and tremulous. Her vital signs are BP 90/60, pulse 100, and temperature 99.8°F.

3. Discuss how M. will be treated for alcohol withdrawal.

4. Identify the symptoms of delirium tremens that the nurse should assess for.

6. You are concerned about M. and her baby. Describe the referrals you will make.

You have observed that M. is a heavy smoker. She has now completed her treatment and is ready to go home.

5. Identify the information that you will give her before discharge.

After delivery, M. plans to start disulfiram (Antabuse).

7. Identify the information that you will provide her.

Study Guide to Accompany Clinical Drug Therapy: Rationales for Nursing Practice, sixth edition, by Gail Ropelewski-Ryan.

CHAPTER 16

Central Nervous System Stimulants

■ Fill in the Blanks

1. Two disorders treated with CNS stimulants are
   _____ and _____.

2. Narcolepsy is _____ by periodic
   "sleep attacks."

3. Attention deficit-hyperactivity disorder (ADHD)
   occurs in _____ and is characterized
   by _____, _____,
   _____, _____, and
   _____.

4. Amphetamines produce _____,
   _____ and _____.
   They also increase _____ and
   _____, produce _____,
   and slow _____. In ADHD these
   drugs also reduce _____ and
   _____.

5. Analeptic drugs stimulate _____. A
   major drawback is the adverse effect of
   _____.

6. Xanthine drugs increase _____ and
   decrease _____.

7. Xanthines also increase _____,
   _____, _____, and
   increase secretion of _____ and
   _____.

8. Methylphenidate (_____) is used for
   children with ADHD. Initially, 5 mg is administered b.i.d. Monday through Friday while children
   are in school. The dose is gradually increased by
   _____ at weekly intervals to a max-
   imum of _____ mg per day.

9. Doxapram (_____) increases tidal
   volume and respiratory rate. Duration of action of
   a single dose is _____ minutes.

10. Caffeine may increase _____. It may
    be combined with ergot alkaloids to treat
    _____.

11. Caffeine and sodium benzoate is used as a respira-
    tory stimulant in _____.

12. Caffeine can produce _____,
    _____, or _____.

13. Children being treated for ADHD should avoid
    _____ in their diet.

14. Dosage adjustments are needed as the child
    _____ and _____ slows.

15. Adverse effects of CNS stimulants in the elderly
    include _____,
    _____, _____ and
    _____.

■ Review Questions

1. A client who is being treated for narcolepsy must be assessed for adverse effects of dextroamphetamine (Dexedrine), which includes
   a. impaired motor coordination.
   b. difficulty concentrating.
   c. muscle atrophy.
   d. altered growth and development.

2. An expected outcome when theophylline is administered is
   a. increased respiratory rate.
   b. increased tidal volume.
   c. bronchodilation.
   d. decreased oxygen demand.

3. When clients are receiving amphetamines, they should be assessed for
   a. weight loss.
   b. decreased urinary output.
   c. decreased pulse rate.
   d. bronchodilation.

4. The expected outcome when doxapram (Dopram) is administered is increased
   a. mental alertness.
   b. respiratory rate.
   c. cardiac output.
   d. oxygen use.

5. An amphetamine overdose can result in
   a. permanent memory loss.
   b. renal failure.
   c. convulsions.
   d. hepatic failure.

6. Which of the following statements by Mr. H. leads you to believe that he has understood the teaching you have done about methylphenidate (Ritalin)?
   a. "Over-the-counter medication has no impact on this medication."
   b. "It produces tolerance, and habituation can occur."
   c. "There are no adverse effects with this medication."
   d. "It should not be taken within 6–8 hours of bedtime."

7. When caffeine is administered with the following drug, it will increase its effect.
   a. Theophylline
   b. Cimetidine (Tagamet)
   c. Propranolol (Inderal)
   d. Furosemide (Lasix)

8. Caffeine is found in all of these over-the-counter medications except
   a. Excedrin.
   b. Vanquish.
   c. No-Doz.
   d. Tylenol.

9. This drug is used as a respiratory stimulant in neonates who are experiencing apnea that is unresponsive to other treatments.
   a. Dextroamphetamine (Dexedrine)
   b. Doxapram (Dopram)
   c. Caffeine and sodium benzoate
   d. Methamphetamine (Desoxyn)

10. The use of central nervous system stimulants is contraindicated in persons with the following disorder.
    a. Depression
    b. Hyperthyroidism
    c. Chronic obstructive pulmonary disease
    d. Diabetes mellitus

CHAPTER 17

Physiology of the Autonomic Nervous System

■ Fill in the Blanks

Use the following terms to fill in the blanks in Table 17-1 on the autonomic nervous system. Each term may be used more than once.

Increases   Decreases   Constricts   Dilates   No effect

■ Table 17–1

AUTONOMIC NERVOUS SYSTEM

Parasympathetic Response	Body Tissue/Organ	Sympathetic Response
1. _____	Blood vessels	8. _____
2. _____ rate	Heart	9. _____ rate
3. _____ contraction		10. _____ contraction
4. _____	Lungs	11. _____
5. _____ sweating	Skin	12. _____ sweating
6. _____	Eye	13. _____
7. _____	Pancreas	14. _____ blood sugar

■ True or False

1. _____ Anticholinergic drugs act by blocking the action of acetylcholine.

2. _____ Cholinergic drugs produce bronchoconstriction.

3. _____ Adrenergic drugs decrease myocardial contractility.

4. _____ Adrenergic drugs may be used in the treatment of tachycardia.

5. _____ Beta-adrenergic blocking agents are given for bronchodilating effects.

6. _____ Beta-blocking drugs may cause tachycardia.

7. _____ The sympathetic nervous system is stimulated by temperature extremes.

8. _____ Dopamine is essential for normal brain function.

■ Review Questions

1. When beta-adrenergic blocking drugs are administered, they increase the person's risk of
   a. tachycardia.
   b. acute myocardial infarction.
   c. hypotension.
   d. atrial fibrillation.

2. An expected outcome with the administration of beta-adrenergic blocking agents is
   a. increased cardiac output.
   b. decreased oxygen consumption.
   c. increased blood pressure.
   d. decreased exercise tolerance.

3. Drugs that stimulate the parasympathetic nervous system cause
   a. decreased sweating.
   b. increased heart rate.
   c. pupillary constriction.
   d. dilation of bronchi.

4. Alpha-adrenergic blocking agents may affect
   a. platelet aggregation.
   b. lipolysis.
   c. release of renin.
   d. glycogenolysis.

5. An agent developed to stimulate beta$_2$ receptors to produce bronchodilation with minimal tachycardia.
   a. Isoproterenol (Isuprel)
   b. Albuterol (Proventil)
   c. Xylometazoline hydrochloride (Otrivin)
   d. Terbutaline (Brethine)

6. When an adrenergic agent is administered, it will
   a. decrease arterial blood pressure.
   b. increase blood sugar.
   c. decrease muscle strength.
   d. increase gastric motility.

7. When anticholinergic agents are administered, the nurse should assess the client for
   a. tachycardia.
   b. diarrhea.
   c. clotting disorders.
   d. hypoglycemia.

8. An expected outcome of the administration of cholinergic drugs is
   a. increased muscle strength.
   b. increased blood pressure.
   c. increased gastric motility.
   d. increased heart rate.

9. A beta-adrenergic blocker should be administered with caution to persons who have this disorder.
   a. Hypertension
   b. Angina
   c. Heart failure
   d. Atrial flutter

10. Which of the following agents inhibit parasympathetic stimulation?
    a. Adrenergic agents
    b. Antiadrenergic agents
    c. Cholinergic agents
    d. Anticholinergic agents

CHAPTER 18

Adrenergic Drugs

■ Matching Exercise

TERMS AND CONCEPTS

Match the concept with the term for it.

1. _____ A drug used for hypotension and shock.

2. _____ An intravenous medication used as a cardiac stimulant to increase the force of the contraction of the heart.

3. _____ This drug produces bronchodilation and increases the heart rate.

4. _____ Commonly used inhaler that produces bronchodilation.

5. _____ This drug is used to relieve the acute brochospasm and laryngeal edema of anaphylatic shock.

6. _____ A drug that decreases the effect of adrenergics.

7. _____ This drug is used for nasal congestion and is found in over-the-counter medication.

8. _____ This substance has a synergistic bronchodilating effect when administered with adrenergic agents.

9. _____ This drug, used for nasal congestion, also acts as an appetite suppressant.

10. _____ Can lose its effectiveness with prolonged use.

A. Isoproterenol (Isuprel)

B. Propranolol (Inderal)

C. Dopamine (Intropin)

D. Dobutamine (Dobutrex)

E. Epinephrine (Adrenalin)

F. Albuterol (Proventil)

G. Caffeine

H. Phenylpropanolamine (Propagest)

I. Pseudoephedrine (Sudafed)

J. Terbutaline (Brethine)

■ True or False

1. _____ Epinephrine (Adrenalin) causes peripheral vasoconstriction and bronchodilation.

2. _____ Common adverse effects from the administration of adrenergic drugs include hypotension and bradycardia.

3. _____ Albuterol (Proventil) should not be given to children under 12 years of age.

4. _____ An expected outcome of the administration of dopamine (Intropin) is increased urinary output.

5. _____ Inhaled solutions of isoproterenol (Isuprel) may turn saliva pink.

6. _____ When nasal decongestants are used excessively, a rebound nasal congestion can result.

7. _____ When adrenergic agents are administered with beta blockers, the effect of the adrenergic agent is increased.

8. _____ Epinephrine (Adrenalin) can only be administered parenterally.

9. _____ A common side effect from the administration of epinephrine (Adrenalin) is elevated serum glucose.

10. _____ The usual goal of vasopressor therapy is to maintain the systolic blood pressure above 80.

■ Sentence Correction

Circle the word that makes the sentence incorrect and place the correct word in the space provided. Example: **increases**
Dobutamine (Dobutrex) (decreases) _cardiac output._

1. _____Ephedrine is used to stimulate the heart and relax bronchial smooth muscle.

2. _____An allergic reaction produces severe respiratory distress and profound hypotension.

3. _____Acute asthma attacks may be precipitated by exposure to toxins.

4. _____Alkalosis may occur with chronic bronchospasm.

5. _____When administering substances known to produce hypersensitivity reactions, observe the recipient carefully for 5 minutes after administration.

6. _____Levarterenol (Levophed) stimulates electrical and mechanical activity to produce myocardial contraction.

7. _____In Stokes-Adams syndrome, adrenergic drugs are given as cardiac depressants.

8. _____Ephedrine is an ingredient in cold medications.

9. _____Isoproterenol (Isuprel) may cause chest pain and bradycardia.

10. _____Isoproterenol (Isuprel) is used to treat both bronchoconstriction and premature labor.

11. _____When giving dopamine (Intropin), observe for improved breathing.

12. _____The use of excessive amounts of nasal decongestants can result in hypotension.

13. _____When assessing for the effectiveness of vasopressors, you should assess blood pressure and the person's respiratory status.

14. _____Anticholinergic drugs decrease the effects of adrenergic drugs.

15. _____Metaraminol (Aramine) is used for bronchodilation and vasoconstriction.

■ Review Questions

1. The use of adrenergic drugs is contraindicated in persons with the following condition.
   a. Diabetes mellitus
   b. Tachycardia
   c. Hypotension
   d. Bronchoconstriction

2. An expected outcome after the administration of dopamine (Intropin) is
   a. increased blood pressure.
   b. headache.
   c. decreased pulse.
   d. decreased respirations.

3. The drug of choice for treating shock due to spinal anesthesia is
   a. ephedrine.
   b. dopamine (Intropin).
   c. dobutamine (Dobutrex).
   d. epinephrine (Adrenalin).

4. Your client has a cardiac arrest and is given epinephrine (Adrenalin). After his condition is stabilized, blood work is drawn and the results are glucose 160, WBC 5000, PTT 15 seconds, potassium 5.0 mEq/L. Which deviation in these lab values is attributable to the use of epinephrine (Adrenalin)?
   a. WBC
   b. Glucose
   c. PTT
   d. Potassium

5. Which of the following comments by Mr. J.'s wife leads you to believe that she has a good understanding of why her husband is receiving terbutaline (Brethine): "The doctor ordered the medication to…"
   a. "increase the force of the contraction of my husband's heart."
   b. "decrease my husband's pCO$_2$."
   c. "improve his oxygen exchange."
   d. "decrease his oxygen requirements."

Study Guide to Accompany Clinical Drug Therapy: Rationales for Nursing Practice, sixth edition, by Gail Ropelewski-Ryan.

6. After a breathing treatment with isoproterenol (Isuprel), your client calls you into her room stating, "My heart is racing; I think something is wrong." Your best response would be
   a. "Lie down and rest and I will take your vital signs in 15 minutes."
   b. "I will contact your physician immediately."
   c. "An increased pulse rate is common when isoproterenol (Isuprel) is given by inhalation."
   d. "You have no need to be alarmed. This is a common side effect."

7. Which of the following medications, if administered concurrently with adrenergic drugs, will decrease their effect?
   a. Beta-adrenergic blockers
   b. Xanthines
   c. Anticholinergics
   d. Tricyclic antidepressants

8. Your client with COPD who is taking albuterol (Proventil) needs to be observed for
   a. anxiety, nervousness, and insomnia.
   b. bradycardia and hypotension.
   c. fluid retention.
   d. bronchoconstriction.

9. Ephedrine works by
   a. stimulating the release of norepinephrine.
   b. blocking beta receptors.
   c. blocking alpha receptors.
   d. stimulating the release of acetylcholine.

10. Epinephrine is used to treat all of the following except
    a. anaphylactic shock.
    b. bronchospasm.
    c. cardiac arrest.
    d. tachycardia.

■ Critical Thinking Case Study

Mr. J. is admitted to the ER because he has an anaphylactic reaction. He is given epinephrine, a corticosteroid, and aminophylline.

1. Explain why these drugs were ordered.

2. Identify what nursing assessments you will be performing and your rationale for each.

3. Explain why antihistamines were not used.

CHAPTER 19

Antiadrenergic Drugs

■ Matching Exercise

TERMS AND CONCEPTS

Match the concept with the term for it.

1. _____ Used for the treatment of supraventricular tachycardia.

2. _____ This drug is valuable in the treatment of glaucoma.

3. _____ A drug of choice for treating hypertensive emergencies.

4. _____ Clients use this drug to prevent migraine headaches.

5. _____ A nonselective beta blocker used to treat glaucoma.

6. _____ This drug is used for prevention of tissue necrosis from extravasation.

7. _____ This drug is effective in treating ventricular arrhythmias.

8. _____ When this drug is administered with beta-adrenergic blockers, heart block can result.

9. _____ An alpha-adrenergic antagonist used for the treatment of hypertension.

10. _____ This drug is administered parenterally for early treatment of myocardial infarction.

A. Labetalol (Trandate)

B. Carteolol (Cartrol)

C. Phentolamine (Regitine)

D. Propranolol (Inderal)

E. Esmolol (Brevibloc)

F. Betaxolol (Betoptic)

G. Digoxin (Lanoxin)

H. Prazosin (Minipress)

I. Acebutolol (Sectral)

J. Metoprolol (Lopressor)

■ True or False

1. _____ A clonidine transdermal patch should be changed daily.

2. _____ Beta blockers act to maximize sympathetic nervous system stimulation of various organs and tissues.

3. _____ Beta blockers decrease the force of myocardial contraction, decrease cardiac output, decrease blood pressure, and decrease heart rate.

4. _____ Beta blockers are apparently equally effective in the treatment of hypertension.

5. _____ Major adverse effects of beta blockers are congestive heart failure, bradycardia, and bronchospasm.

6. _____ Adverse effects of beta-adrenergic blockers include CNS problems (eg, nervousness, insomnia, hallucinations, mental depression) and sexual dysfunction (eg, impotence, decreased libido).

7. _____ Metoprolol (Lopressor), atenolol (Tenormin), and acebutolol (Sectral) are cardioselective.

8. _____ Propranolol (Inderal) is used in the treatment of hypertension, angina pectoris, and cardiac dysrhythmias.

9. _____ Atenolol (Tenormin), metoprolol (Lopressor), propranolol (Inderal), and timolol (Blocadren) are approved for use in prevention of reinfarction.

10. _____ Beta blockers are used to treat frostbite.

■ Fill in the Blanks

Fill in the blanks in Figure 19-1 with the terms below.

Myocardial or other tissue cells

Beta-adrenergic blocking drugs

Epinephrine and norepinephrine

Nerve endings

Receptor site

FIGURE 19-1

■ Sentence Correction

Circle the word that makes the sentence incorrect and place the correct word in the space provided. Example:
Esmolol (Brevibloc) *Propranolol is used to treat supraventricular tachycardia.*

1. _____ Nadolol (Corgard) is the oldest of the beta-blocking agents.

2. _____ Acebutolol (Sectral) is a nonselective beta blocker used to treat hypertension.

3. _____ Esmolol (Brevibloc) is the drug of choice for treating hypertension.

4. _____ A nonselective beta blocker used to treat glaucoma is pindolol (Visken).

5. _____ The beta blocker of choice for treating migraine headaches is levobunolol (Betagan).

6. _____ Metoprolol (Lopressor) is an alpha blocker used for the treatment of benign prostatic hypertrophy.

7. _____ A cardioselective beta block-er used for the treatment of angina is penbutolol (Levatol).

8. _____ Selective beta blockers should not be used for persons with respiratory diseases.

9. _____ A nonselective beta blocker used for the treatment of a myocardial infarction is levobunolol (Betagan).

10. _____ Beta-adrenergic blocking agents are used when the individual has had a stroke.

11. _____ Timolol (Timoptic) reduces intraocular pressure by increasing the formation of aqueous humor.

12. _____ The term "selective" indi-cates that those drugs have more effect on beta$_2$ receptors.

13. _____ Beta blockers are likely to cause tachycardia.

14. _____ Beta blockers that are highly water soluble are more likely to cause depression, nightmares, insomnia, and hallucinations.

15. _____ In the presence of hepatic disease, the dosage of timolol should be increased.

■ Review Questions

1. Mr. P. has hypertension and a ventricular dys-rhythmia. Which of the following beta-adrenergic blocking agents would be most effective for him?
   a. Acebutolol (Sectral)
   b. Atenolol (Tenormin)
   c. Esmolol (Brevibloc)
   d. Metoprolol (Lopressor)

2. Which of the following beta-adrenergic blocking agents would be most effective in treating supraventricular tachycardia?
   a. Propranolol (Inderal)
   b. Nadolol (Corgard)
   c. Esmolol (Brevibloc)
   d. Acebutolol (Sectral)

3. Alpha$_2$-adrenergic agonist agents will
   a. increase sodium retention.
   b. decrease insulin secretion.
   c. increase cardiac output.
   d. decrease oxygen consumption.

4. Mr. C. is receiving propranolol (Inderal) for migraine headaches. It is important to assess Mr. C.'s pulse rate and to examine his lab studies for a possible drop in
   a. serum potassium.
   b. WBC.
   c. blood sugar.
   d. hemoglobin.

5. Which of the following statements by Mrs. H. leads you to believe that she understands the teaching that you have done regarding atenolol (Tenormin)?
   a. "If I experience side effects, I will stop taking the medication."
   b. "I am not allowed to have any caffeine."
   c. "Smoking will not reduce the effectiveness of the medication."
   d. "I will take my pulse daily."

6. Which of the following drugs, when administered with propranolol (Inderal), will decrease the effect of Inderal?
   a. Atropine
   b. Digoxin (Lanoxin)
   c. Phenytoin (Dilantin)
   d. Quinidine

7. Which of the following instructions should be included when you are discharging a client on metoprolol (Lopressor)?
   a. "When taking this drug, you should exercise strenuously 30 minutes a day."
   b. "Report weight loss of more than 2 lb in 1 week."
   c. "Take the medication on an empty stomach to enhance its absorption."
   d. "Ingestion of alcohol with this drug can cause dizziness."

8. In reviewing Mr. J.'s history, you discover that he has a history of diabetes mellitus, myocardial infarction, multiple sclerosis, and peptic ulcer disease. Which one of these diagnoses would you discuss with the physician before administering a beta-adrenergic blocker?

   a. Myocardial infarction

   b. Multiple sclerosis

   c. Diabetes mellitus

   d. Peptic ulcer disease

9. When a nonselective beta blocker is administered, there is a greater risk of

   a. bronchoconstriction.

   b. reflex tachycardia.

   c. respiratory depression.

   d. arrhythmias.

10. Which of the following beta blockers has been approved to treat heart failure?

   a. Atenolol (Tenormin)

   b. Nadolol (Corgard)

   c. Carteolol (Cartrol)

   d. Carvedilol (Coreg)

■ Critical Thinking Case Study

Your client, Mrs. M., is a 54-year-old woman diagnosed with essential hypertension. Her blood pressure is 140/90. Her physician places her on nadolol (Corgard).

1. Identify the teaching you will do with Mrs. M. that will help her control her hypertension.

2. Identify the concurrent medical diagnosis that would preclude the use of Corgard.

After 2 months, Mrs. M. returns. Her blood pressure is still elevated, and her physician adds Hydrodiuril to her regimen.

3. Identify the rationale for the multiple-drug regimen.

Discuss the adverse effects associated with each medication.

4. Identify the objective assessments that will be important when monitoring Mrs. M.

CHAPTER 20

Cholinergic Drugs

■ Fill in the Blanks

Use the following terms to fill in the blanks. Each term may be used more than once.

Increased   Decreased

Relaxation of   Constriction of

1. Direct-acting cholinergic drugs cause
   a. _____ heart rate.
   b. _____ contractility of gastrointestinal smooth muscle.
   c. _____ sphincters.
   d. _____ contractility of smooth muscle of the bladder.
   e. _____ contractility of bronchial smooth muscle.
   f. _____ respiratory secretions.
   g. _____ pupils.

■ Matching Exercise

TERMS AND CONCEPTS

Match the drug with its action.

1. _____ Bethanechol (Urecholine)

2. _____ Neostigmine (Prostigmin)

3. _____ Edrophonium (Tensilon)

4. _____ Tacrine (Cognex)

5. _____ Physostigmine salicylate (Antilirium)

A. Used as an antidote for tubocurarine.

B. Used to diagnose myasthenia gravis.

C. Used to treat Alzheimer's disease.

D. Used for urinary retention and paralytic ileus.

E. Used as an antidote for "atropine poisoning."

■ True or False

1. _____ With myasthenia gravis, the dosage of anticholinesterase drugs may need to be increased if the client develops an infection.

2. _____ Bethanechol (Urecholine) should not be administered IM or IV.

3. _____ Hypertension is a common side effect of cholinergic drugs.

4. _____ When antihistamines are administered concurrently with cholinergic drugs, they decrease the effect of the cholinergic drug.

5. _____ Pyridostigmine (Mestinon) is taken at bedtime to prevent the client from experiencing an inability to swallow upon awakening.

■ Review Questions

1. Your client asks you why his physician ordered bethanechol (Urecholine) for him postoperatively. The best response is to explain that bethanechol is administered postoperatively to
   a. improve gastric motility.
   b. decrease adventitious breath sounds.
   c. decrease abdominal discomfort.
   d. increase urinary output.

2. An expected outcome after administration of pyridostigmine for myasthenia gravis is
   a. improved appetite.
   b. fewer headaches.
   c. increased muscle strength.
   d. decreased tremors.

3. The physician has ordered neostigmine (Prostigmin) for a client with paraplegia to
   a. increase bladder capacity.
   b. increase urinary output.
   c. increase muscle strength.
   d. prevent constipation.

4. Which of the following anticholinergic drugs is the drug of choice for a tubocurarine overdose?
   a. Bethanechol (Urecholine)
   b. Neostigmine (Prostigmin)
   c. Edrophonium (Tensilon)
   d. Physostigmine salicylate (Antilirium)

5. Which of the following statements by your client leads you to believe that she has understood the teaching you have done regarding pyridostigmine (Mestinon)?
   a. "I will limit my fluid intake to 1500 cc while I am taking this medication."
   b. "If I have increased sweating, I will contact the doctor immediately."
   c. "It is important that I take this medication on time."
   d. "I will take the medication with meals."

6. The antidote the physician should have on hand when he or she is administering edrophonium (Tensilon) is
   a. atropine.
   b. dopamine (Intropin).
   c. phenytoin (Dilantin).
   d. epinephrine.

7. When you are administering bethanechol (Urecholine) to Mr. B., you should observe him for evidence of a cholinergic crisis. Symptoms include
   a. hypertension.
   b. confusion.
   c. fever.
   d. respiratory failure.

8. For which of the following disorders is the use of cholinergics contraindicated?
   a. Hypertension
   b. Parkinson's disease
   c. Diabetes mellitus
   d. Peptic ulcer disease

9. An adverse effect after administration of cholinergic agents is increased
   a. heart rate.
   b. serum glucose level.
   c. blood pressure.
   d. respiratory secretions.

10. Which of the following instructions should you give Mr. G., who is starting on bethanechol (Urecholine)?
    a. "Avoid foods high in vitamin C."
    b. "Increase your fluid intake to 3000 cc a day."
    c. "Increase the roughage in your diet."
    d. "Take the medication before meals."

■ Critical Thinking Case Study

J., a 9-year-old boy weighing 66 lb, is admitted to your unit following surgery for a ruptured appendix. He has an NG tube to suction intermittently and a Foley catheter in place. No bowel sounds are auscultated. (The learner may need to use additional sources to answer the questions.)

1. Discuss why it is common for there to be no bowel sounds after abdominal surgery, and when you can expect bowel sounds to return.

2. Identify the electrolyte imbalances you should assess for.

Three days after surgery, J.'s abdomen is distended. He has only faint hypoactive bowel sounds and is having difficulty voiding. The physician orders bethanechol (Urecholine) 5 mg q.i.d.

3. Identify why the physician ordered this medication and whether the dose the physician ordered is within the therapeutic range for J.

You go into J.'s room to administer his morning dose of bethanechol (Urecholine) and find that his pupils are constricted. His pulse is 110, respirations 16, BP 80/60, and temperature 102°F. J. complains of a headache and nausea. You notice that his bed is wet from perspiration.

5. Identify which signs and symptoms from your assessment are directly related to the cholinergic drug he is taking, and what your nursing actions will be.

4. Identify the expected outcome after this medication is administered.

J. becomes short of breath.

6. Identify and prioritize your nursing actions.

CHAPTER 21

Anticholinergic Drugs

■ Fill in the Blanks

Complete the following sentences.

1. Anticholinergic drugs block the action of
   _____ on the _____
   nervous system.

2. The effects that anticholinergic drugs have on the
   body include

   a. _____

   b. _____

   c. _____

   d. _____

   e. _____

   f. _____

   g. _____

   h. _____

3. GI disorders for which anticholinergics are useful
   include _____,
   _____, _____,
   _____, _____, and
   _____.

4. Anticholinergics are used in ophthalmology to aid
   in _____ or _____
   because they produce _____ and
   _____ effects.

5. Atropine is given to _____ the heart
   rate.

6. When a client has chronic bronchoconstriction,
   ipratropium (Atrovent) may be given by
   _____.

7. In Parkinson's disease, anticholinergic drugs are
   used to _____, _____
   and _____.

8. Atropine and glycopyrrolate (Robinul) are used
   preoperatively to reduce _____ and
   _____.

9. Contraindications for the use of anticholinergic
   drugs include _____,
   _____, _____,
   _____, _____,
   _____, and _____
   unless bradycardia is present.

10. Atropine is the _____ anticholiner-
    gic drug and can be administered
    _____, _____,
    _____, _____,
    _____, and by _____.

11. Hyoscyamine (Anaspaz) is a belladonna alkaloid
    used for gastrointestinal and urinary tract disor-
    ders that cause _____,
    _____, and _____.

12. Scopolamine is also used for _____.
    It can be administered orally and as a
    _____, which is effective for
    _____ hours.

13. _____ (Artane) is used for initial
    treatment of _____. It is also effec-
    tive in treating _____ caused by
    antipsychotic drugs.

14. _____ (Cogentin) is used for pre-
    vention and treatment of _____.

15. Flavoxate (Urispas) relieves _____,
    _____, _____, and
    _____.

16. Oxybutynin (_____) increases _____ and decreases _____.

17. Anticholinergic drugs are used to treat

    a. _____

    b. _____

    c. _____

    d. _____

    e. _____

    f. _____

18. The antidote for an atropine overdose is _____ (_____).

19. Adverse responses to anticholinergic agents seen in children include _____ and _____.

20. Common adverse reactions from anticholinergic drugs that the elderly experience include _____, _____, _____, _____, _____, _____, and _____.

■ True or False

1. _____ Meperidine (Demerol) and atropine cannot be mixed in the same syringe.

2. _____ Saunas should be avoided by persons taking anticholinergic drugs.

3. _____ Anticholinergic drugs are used to produce pupillary constriction.

4. _____ Persons taking anticholinergics for peptic ulcer disease should also drink large amounts of milk to decrease gastric acid secretion.

5. _____ Dental caries and loss of teeth can occur from decreased saliva production due to administration of anticholinergic drugs.

■ Matching Exercise

Match the generic and trade names of the anticholinergic drugs.

1. _____ Urispas

2. _____ Cogentin

3. _____ Artane

4. _____ Anaspaz

5. _____ Pamine

6. _____ Robinul

A. Trihexyphenidyl

B. Hyoscyamine

C. Flavoxate

D. Benztropine

E. Methscopolamine

F. Glycopyrrolate

■ Review Questions

1. A client asks you why his physician ordered atropine for him preoperatively. Your best response is to explain that atropine is administered preoperatively to

    a. prevent hypertension.

    b. decrease adventitious breath sounds.

    c. decrease respiratory tract secretions.

    d. increase urinary output.

2. An expected outcome after administration of trihexyphenidyl (Artane) for Parkinson's disease is

    a. improved appetite.

    b. fewer headaches.

    c. a regular gait.

    d. decreased tremors.

3. Persons taking anticholinergic medications are susceptible to heat exhaustion and should do the following to minimize that risk.

    a. Eat a diet high in sodium.

    b. Exercise 30 minutes a day in the morning or evening.

    c. Take cool baths and wear cool clothing.

    d. Avoid going outside.

4. Mr. J. is started on trihexyphenidyl (Artane) for treatment of Parkinson's disease. Which of the following instructions should he be given?

   a. "This medication should be taken once a day at bedtime."

   b. "Take this medication on an empty stomach."

   c. "You may experience mouth dryness from this medication."

   d. "This medication will stop the progression of the disease."

5. Mrs. G. is having extrapyramidal symptoms caused by the phenothiazines she is taking. Which of the following anticholinergic agents would be most effective in treating her symptoms?

   a. Glycopyrrolate (Robinul)

   b. Hyoscyamine (Anaspaz)

   c. Methscopolamine (Pamine)

   d. Trihexyphenidyl (Artane)

6. Anticholinergics are given to increase bladder capacity in clients who have

   a. bladder spasms.

   b. chronic urinary tract infections.

   c. indwelling catheters.

   d. enuresis.

7. Which of the following medications would be most effective in treating an atropine overdose?

   a. Physostigmine salicylate (Antilirium)

   b. Dopamine (Intropin)

   c. Phenytoin (Dilantin)

   d. Epinephrine

8. Inadvertently, your client was given two preoperative injections of Demerol 100 mg IM and atropine 0.25 mg IM. Which of the following adverse reactions is most likely to occur as a result of an atropine overdose?

   a. Increased respiratory secretions

   b. Heat stroke and vomiting

   c. Urinary retention and decreased intestinal motility

   d. Hypotension and bradycardia

9. An expected outcome after administration of high doses of atropine is

   a. increased heart rate.

   b. elevated blood glucose level.

   c. decreased blood pressure.

   d. increased respiratory rate.

10. After receiving atropine, Mrs. J. complains of eye pain. You know that this may be indicative of

    a. a common harmless reaction to the medication.

    b. increased intraocular pressure.

    c. excessive CNS stimulation.

    d. CNS depression.

■ Critical Thinking Case Study

Mr. P., a 76-year-old man with heart failure, is brought to the hospital because he fainted at home. He has been taking digoxin (Lanoxin), furosemide (Lasix), and KCl (potassium chloride) for 5 years. He is alert and oriented but weak. When you check Mr. P.'s apical pulse, you find it to be 40. The physician diagnoses heart block and administers atropine. Soon after the administration of atropine, Mr. P. becomes agitated and confused. (The learner may need to use additional sources to answer the questions.)

1. Identify and prioritize your nursing actions.

Mr. P. is complaining of a dry mouth and blurred vision.

2. Describe your response to Mr. P.

Mr. P.'s physician decides to insert a pacemaker. Mr. P. states, "Now I will no longer need to take medication for my heart failure."

3. Specify the best response.

Study Guide to Accompany Clinical Drug Therapy: Rationales for Nursing Practice, sixth edition, by Gail Ropelewski-Ryan.

CHAPTER 22

Physiology of the Endocrine System

■ Matching Exercise

TERMS AND CONCEPTS

Match the concept with the term for it.

1. _____ Helps maintain fluid balance.

2. _____ Influence carbohydrate storage.

3. _____ Promote sodium retention and potassium loss.

4. _____ The adrenal medulla secretes this hormone.

5. _____ These hormones regulate the metabolic rate of the body.

6. _____ This hormone regulates calcium and phosphate metabolism.

7. _____ Regulates the metabolism of glucose, lipids, and proteins.

8. _____ Promotes the development of secondary sex characteristics in females.

9. _____ Regulates the development of male secondary sex characteristics.

10. _____ Helps prepare the mammary glands for lactation.

11. _____ Stimulates bone marrow to produce RBCs.

12. _____ A hormone that is important in digestion.

13. _____ A hormone secreted in 24-hour cycles

A. Parathyroid hormone

B. Glucagon

C. Testicular hormone

D. ADH

E. Glucocorticoids

F. Mineralocorticoids

G. Estrogen

H. Progesterone

I. Epinephrine

J. Thyroid hormones

K. Gastrin

L. Erythropoietin

M. ACTH

■ True or False

1. _____ The length of the physiologic effects of the endocrine hormones varies from minutes to hours.

2. _____ Secretion of hormones is controlled by the thalamus.

3. _____ Cancerous tumors can produce hormones.

4. _____ Steroid hormones are synthesized from amino acids.

5. _____ Secretion of all pituitary hormones is controlled by the hypothalamus.

6. _____ Estrogen and progestin are secreted in 24-hour cycles.

7. _____ Angiotensin II is a strong vasoconstrictor that controls blood pressure.

8. _____ Steroid hormones are water soluble and cross the cell membrane easily.

■ Review Questions

1. Along with insulin, the pancreatic hormone that helps regulate the metabolism of glucose is
   a. epinephrine.
   b. lactogen.
   c. cortisol.
   d. glucagon.

2. The secretion of pituitary hormone is controlled by the
   a. hypothalamus.
   b. anterior pituitary.
   c. posterior pituitary.
   d. thalamus.

3. The antidiuretic hormone is released in response to
   a. increased blood pressure.
   b. increased serum sodium levels.
   c. decreased plasma protein.
   d. increased blood pressure.

4. ADH is secreted by the
   a. anterior pituitary.
   b. posterior pituitary.
   c. thyroid gland.
   d. parathyroid gland.

5. Mineralocorticoids help regulate
   a. electrolyte balance.
   b. metabolism of glucose, lipids, and proteins.
   c. the development of feminine characteristics.
   d. carbohydrate storage and protein catabolism.

6. Adrenal medulla hormones that affect the heart rate and blood pressure are
   a. cortisol and aldosterone.
   b. gastrin and enterogastrone.
   c. secretin and cholecystokinin.
   d. epinephrine and norepinephrine.

7. An insulin-dependent diabetic is started on a glucocorticoid. The addition of this medication
   a. will have no effect on his insulin requirements.
   b. may increase his insulin requirements.
   c. may decrease his insulin requirements.
   d. is likely to cause a toxic effect that must be carefully assessed for.

8. Your client's parathyroid gland was inadvertently removed during surgery. You should assess him for
   a. respiratory distress.
   b. tetany.
   c. hypertension.
   d. sodium retention.

9. Erythropoietin
   a. stimulates the bone marrow to produce RBCs.
   b. stimulates the growth of bones and muscles.
   c. regulates the osmolality of extracellular fluids.
   d. promotes sodium and water retention.

10. A type 2 diabetic is reluctant to start on insulin. Your best response would be
    a. "Insulin helps regulate the metabolism of glucose, something that your body is no longer able to do."
    b. "Insulin helps regulate the growth of bone and muscle cells and will prevent you from getting fractures in the future."
    c. "Insulin raises blood glucose levels by promoting the breakdown of glycogen in the liver; without the medication, this would not be possible."
    d. "Insulin regulates the osmolality of the extracellular fluid. Without insulin, you would retain fluid."

CHAPTER 23

Hypothalamic and Pituitary Hormones

■ Matching Exercise

TERMS AND CONCEPTS

Match the concept with the term for it.

1. _____ The posterior pituitary.

2. _____ Stimulates functions of sex glands.

3. _____ Plays a role in skin pigmentation.

4. _____ Plays a part in milk production in nursing mothers.

5. _____ Also called vasopressin.

6. _____ Excessive production of this hormone can result in giantism.

7. _____ Drug used in treatment of diabetes insipidus.

8. _____ Drug used to induce labor.

9. _____ Drug used to induce ovulation.

10. _____ Drug used as a diagnostic test in suspected adrenal insufficiency.

11. _____ Sudden discontinuation of this drug may cause weakness, fatigue, and hypotension.

12. _____ Drug used in the treatment of endometriosis.

13. _____ Inhibits the release of growth hormone.

14. _____ Causes the release of TSH in response to stress.

15. _____ Used for carcinoid tumors to inhibit diarrhea.

A. Follicle-stimulating hormone (FSH)

B. Oxytocin (Pitocin)

C. Menotropins (Pergonal)

D. Melanocyte-stimulating hormone

E. Cosyntropin (Cortrosyn)

F. Neurohypophysis

G. Lypressin

H. Antidiuretic hormone (ADH)

I. Prolactin

J. Corticotropin (ACTH)

K. Nafarelin (Synarel)

L. Growth hormone

M. Octreotide (Sandostatin)

N. Thyrotropin-releasing hormone (TRH)

O. Somatostatin

■ Fill in the Blanks

Fill in the blanks in the chart with the terms listed below to describe pituitary function.

ACTH   Oxytocin   Growth hormone

FSH   TSH   LH

Prolactin   ADH

Anterior Pituitary

1. _____
   Stimulates secretion of milk

2. _____
   Regulates body growth

3. _____
   Regulates thyroid gland
   activity

4. _____
   Regulates activity of the
   adrenal cortex

5. _____
   Female:
   Stimulates ovulation
   and luteinization
   Male:
   Stimulates spermatogenesis

6. _____
   Female:
   Stimulates growth and activity
   of ovarian follicles
   Male:
   Stimulates growth of seminifer-
   ous tubules and spermatogenesis

Posterior Pituitary

7. _____
   Promotes retention of water
   (reduces urinary volume)

8. _____
   Contracts muscle in wall
   of uterus

■ Review Questions

1. Your client is being treated for adrenal dysfunction. You know that she understands the teaching
   you have done regarding corticotropin (ACTH) if
   she states the following:
   a. "I will not drink more than 1500 mL daily."
   b. "I will avoid excessive exposure to the sun."
   c. "I will weigh myself weekly and report a
      weight loss of more than 2 lb."
   d. "I will eat foods low in sodium and high in
      potassium."

2. You should contact the physician if you observe
   which of the following adverse effects during the
   administration of vasopressin (Pitressin)?
   a. Bradycardia
   b. Coughing
   c. Chest pain
   d. Diarrhea

3. The nurse should instruct a client who is taking
   corticotropin (ACTH) that abrupt withdrawal of
   the drug can result in
   a. confusion, lethargy, and hypertension.
   b. nausea, vomiting, and diarrhea.
   c. headache, dizziness, and blurred vision.
   d. weakness, fatigue, and hypotension.

4. C.J. is receiving somatropin (Humatrope) because
   of a growth deficiency. Which of the following lab
   studies should be done on a regular basis?
   a. WBC
   b. Serum glucose levels
   c. Hemoglobin
   d. Serum potassium levels

5. Which of the following medications, if administered with vasopressin, would decrease its effect?

a. Estrogen

b. Lithium carbonate (Eskalith)

c. Cosyntropin (Cortrosyn)

d. Chlorpropamide (Diabinese)

6. Oxytocin (Pitocin), when administered rapidly to a woman in labor, can cause

a. respiratory distress.

b. uterine spasms.

c. cardiac arrest.

d. renal shut down.

7. An expected outcome after administration of desmopressin (Stimate) is decreased

a. blood pressure.

b. serum potassium levels.

c. specific gravity.

d. urinary output.

8. When administering lypressin, the most important assessment is

a. breath sounds.

b. apical pulse.

c. blood pressure.

d. output.

9. Somatropin (Humatrope) should be administered to children with growth impairment before

a. age 2.

b. entering school.

c. puberty.

d. age 18.

10. Mr. J. is admitted with a carcinoid tumor and is experiencing continuous diarrrhea. An effective treatment for this problem is

a. octreotide (Sandostatin).

b. Lomotil.

c. nafarelin (Synarel).

d. Metamucil.

■ Critical Thinking Case Study

Ms. G., an 18-year-old primigravida, has been in labor for 6 hours and her labor is not progressing. Her physician decides to start an oxytocin (Pitocin) drip.

1. Explain to Ms. G. the rationale for starting this medication and what she can expect.

2. Identify your nursing responsibilities.

The order for the oxytocin (Pitocin) reads: 1–2 milliunits/min; increase by 1–2 milliunits every 15 minutes.

3. Discuss why the medication is administered in this way.

Two hours after starting the oxytocin (Pitocin), Ms. G. starts screaming, "I can't take the pain; do something!"

4. Identify and prioritize your nursing actions.

Ms. G. delivers a 9 lb, 6 oz healthy baby boy. After delivery, the physician wants the oxytocin (Pitocin) drip continued. Ms. G. starts crying and says, "Why can't they stop the medication now that I've had the baby?"

5. Identify your best response.

Study Guide to Accompany Clinical Drug Therapy: Rationales for Nursing Practice, sixth edition, by Gail Ropelewski-Ryan.

CHAPTER 24

Corticosteroids

■ True or False

1. _____ Secretion of corticosteroids normally decreases during periods of stress.

2. _____ Secretion of corticosteroids is normally controlled by a positive feedback mechanism.

3. _____ Endogenous corticosteroids are those obtained from a source outside the human body.

4. _____ Glucocorticoids promote wound healing.

5. _____ Glucocorticoids may cause hyperglycemia and diabetes mellitus as a result of increased production and decreased use of glucose.

6. _____ Glucocorticoids are often given therapeutically for anti-inflammatory effects.

7. _____ Aldosterone conserves water and sodium and eliminates potassium.

8. _____ Sex hormones are produced by the adrenal glands of both men and women.

9. _____ Corticosteroid drugs cure the diseases for which they are given.

10. _____ A major adverse effect of corticosteroid drug therapy is suppression of the HPA axis.

11. _____ Glucocorticoid therapy can precipitate gastrointestinal bleeding.

12. _____ Long-term corticosteroid drug therapy should be reserved for life-threatening conditions or severe, disabling symptoms that do not respond to other measures.

13. _____ The dosage of corticosteroids must be tapered slowly when the drug is discontinued.

14. _____ Alternate day therapy is used for children receiving corticosteroids so it does not affect their growth.

15. _____ When corticosteroids are being used for adrenal insufficiency, they should be administered between 6 PM and 9 PM.

16. _____ Persons using corticosteroids may need potassium supplementation.

17. _____ Osteoporosis is an adverse effect of long-term corticosteroid therapy.

18. _____ Acne is effectively treated with steroids.

■ Checklist

UNDESIRABLE EFFECTS OF DRUG ADMINISTRATION

Place a check mark beside the words or phrases that indicate adverse effects of corticosteroid drug therapy.

1. _____ Dehydration
2. _____ Rounded or "moon" face
3. _____ Hyperglycemia
4. _____ Delayed wound healing
5. _____ Edema
6. _____ Inhibition of bone growth
7. _____ Oliguria
8. _____ Protein depletion
9. _____ Hypertension
10. _____ Tissue wasting
11. _____ Impaired ability to cope with stress
12. _____ Euphoria
13. _____ Cushing's disease
14. _____ Hypernatremia
15. _____ Hypercorticism
16. _____ Nausea and vomiting
17. _____ Change in sleep patterns
18. _____ Diarrhea
19. _____ Excessive sweating
20. _____ Depression
21. _____ Personality changes
22. _____ Increased intraocular pressure
23. _____ Anorexia
24. _____ Peptic ulcer disease

■ Word Scramble

Provide the trade name for each generic name, then circle the trade name in the word find.

1. beclomethasone _____
2. betamethasone _____
3. fludrocortisone _____
4. flunisolide _____
5. triamcinolone hexacetonide _____
6. hydrocortisone _____
7. methylprednisolone _____
8. prednisolone _____
9. cortisone _____
10. fluticasone _____
11. dexamethasone _____
12. triamcinolone _____
13. prednisolone sodium phosphate _____
14. prednisone _____

■ Review Questions

1. The corticosteroid of choice for treating cerebral edema is
   a. triamcinolone acetonide (Azmacort).
   b. betamethasone (Celestone).
   c. cortisone (Cortone).
   d. dexamethasone (Decadron).

2. Administration of corticosteroids causes
   a. sodium to be excreted.
   b. potassium to be excreted.
   c. potassium to be reabsorbed.
   d. hydrogen to be reabsorbed.

3. You are admitting 65-year-old Mr. J., who is to receive methylprednisolone sodium succinate (Solu-Medrol) for asthma. For which of the following diseases should steroids be administered with caution?
   a. Peripheral vascular disease
   b. Prostatic hypertrophy
   c. Chronic obstructive pulmonary disease
   d. Peptic ulcer disease

```
A P P L H E X N O T H S B H Y P O F T I L C L C E
B F G H D J K A D R E N E R G I C E N B E C T A Z
C O L A E N E C M R A I S S A N L L X Q K O V Z S
D E A N L V C D N C H T N H X Y Z T I P L R D N E
E G G H T D R O E O N I R Y L A R N V R H T L P O
F O N T A D I L N C A Y Y D O D A V P P J O F N V
A N L E S C B R E I K X F E H T G N A E B N O S B
R I F L O R I N E F L U A L A C A A I D A E U K L
O E E U N R E T O R P M X T T O S H R F R N O H A
Y P X C E L E S T O N E D R K B B L K A O T L R N
A J R E C L N O N O T D H A R I S T O C O R T S B
H Y P O F T I L C L C R E S F G H H J N K K A D R
E N E R G I C E L N B O E O T D A Z O L O L A N E
C M R A I S S I A N E L L L X E K V Z S X C W C A
H L P O D I R L A U D I D N A C A Y Y O D A U P J
R I L U A E C A A I D A V H A L D R O N X H A P
D K B E C L A O T L R N A Y J D R E C L N O S T Y
M P E N A M B E R E C V A S G R O N I Q P P F E N
T A A E R O B I D N Y L K I G O N L O K C T K X T
G V A A N G A R I S T O S P A N T A P E S C O R N
I U O U S A L E T M O D T I I B T U D H T R P P L
A S O N B S O R P H Y D R O C O C O R T E F I O N
C W A C I N U C N K I X O P T O R I T A R N G I N
Y B P I X K U N L S I N E T A X A A Y B A I D L E
S F N D N S V D F H C I A N I G E M O R N P H A N
K O N M F L O N A S E E G D E P E R R T E S P L O
```

4. Your client is being treated with cortisone (Cortone). You know the drug is effective if there is a decrease in the symptoms of adrenal insufficiency, which include

   a. anxiety, restlessness, and insomnia.

   b. diarrhea, tachycardia, and hypertension.

   c. weakness, anorexia, and hypotension.

   d. hyperglycemia, hypernatremia, and hypokalemia.

5. Your client has type 2 diabetes, and is to be started on prednisone (Deltasone) for arthritis. You should be aware of the potential for

   a. decreased blood glucose levels.

   b. increased serum potassium levels.

   c. decreased effectiveness of prednisone.

   d. increased blood glucose levels.

6. You know that your client, who is taking cortisone acetate (Cortone) for arthritis, understands the discharge teaching you have done if he states

   a. "I will stop the medicine if I become nauseated."

   b. "I will use aspirin-containing products as needed."

   c. "I will take my medication with an antacid to prevent GI irritation."

   d. "I will have my blood pressure checked daily."

7. Which of the following medications, if administered with corticosteroids, will decrease their effect?

   a. Insulin

   b. Estrogen

   c. Amitriptyline (Elavil)

   d. Phenytoin (Dilantin)

8. Which of the following medications, when administered with corticosteroids, will increase their effect?

   a. Salicylates

   b. Antihistamines

   c. Barbiturates

   d. Anticholinergic agents

9. Dosages of corticosteroids need to be reduced if the following condition is present.

   a. Adrenal insufficiency

   b. Diarrhea

   c. Hyperthyroidism

   d. Hypoalbuminemia

10. G.P., age 9, is receiving prednisone along with other immunosuppressants to prevent rejection of his newly transplanted kidney. It is important for you to give G.P.'s parents which of the following instructions?

   a. "Stunting of growth can occur with long-term steroid use."

   b. "Long-term steroid use can prevent development of secondary sexual characteristics."

   c. "Long-term steroid use can cause weight loss."

   d. "Alopecia can occur with long-term steroid use."

■ Critical Thinking Case Study

G., age 9, is started on prednisone for glomerulonephritis because he has begun spilling protein into his urine.

1. Identify the instructions you will give G.'s mother before he goes home.

G.'s mother asks you what she can expect in terms of length of treatment, ongoing tests, and the like.

2. Describe how you will respond to her questions.

You see G.'s mother 6 months later and she is crying. She states that G. has gained 15 lb, and that the children at school are making fun of her son and he is very unhappy.

3. Identify the best response to G.'s mother, including any suggestions that would be helpful.

CHAPTER 25

Thyroid and Antithyroid Drugs

■ Fill in the Blanks

Complete the following sentences.

1. Production of T_3 and T_4 depends on the presence of _____.

2. Thyroid hormone controls _____, thereby influencing _____.

3. Thyroid hormones are required for _____ and _____.

4. Symptoms of hypothyroidism in children include _____, _____, _____, _____, _____, _____, and _____.

5. The symptoms of adult hypothyroidism are _____.

6. A person with hyperthyroidism will exhibit these CNS effects: _____, _____, _____, _____, _____, and _____.

7. Thyroid storm or thyrotoxic crisis is characterized by _____, _____, _____, _____, and _____.

8. Hyperthyroidism is treated with _____, _____, or _____.

9. The drug of choice for treating hypothyroidism is _____, and it is administered _____. The usual maintenance dose is _____ daily.

10. Propylthiouracil (Propacil) is used to treat _____.

11. SSKI (Saturated Solution of Potassium Iodide) is used as an _____ but may also be given _____.

12. An antiadrenergic drug used to treat cardiovascular conditions associated with hyperthyroidism is _____ (_____). It is used to control the following symptoms associated with excessive SNS stimulation _____, _____, _____, _____, and _____.

13. The normal value for TSH is _____.

14. Antithyroid drugs are administered for _____ months.

15. Children who are receiving thyroid replacement should have the following parameters monitored regularly: _____ and _____.

16. In older adults, levothyroxine (Synthroid) should be held if the resting HR is greater than _____.

■ Nursing Diagnosis

S., age 5, is taken to the pediatrician for her school physical and hyperthyroidism is discovered. Identify three possible nursing diagnoses, pertinent assessment data, and nursing interventions associated with hyperthyroidism.

1. Nursing Diagnosis:

   Assessment Data:

   Nursing Interventions:

2. Nursing Diagnosis:

   Assessment Data:

   Nursing Interventions:

3. Nursing Diagnosis:

   Assessment Data:

   Nursing Interventions:

■ Definitions

Define the following terms.

1. Goiter _____

   _____

2. Cretinism _____

   _____

3. Myxedema _____

   _____

4. Thyroid storm _____

   _____

■ Review Questions

1. After a thyroidectomy, your client is placed on Synthroid. Which of the following statements would indicate that your client has understood the teaching you have done?

   a. "I can expect to feel tired and nauseated initially."

   b. "I will monitor my weight and pulse regularly."

   c. "When my symptoms subside, I will no longer need medication."

   d. "I can continue to use over-the-counter cold preparations."

2. Mr. J. has blood work done. His T_3 is 0.08 and T_4 is 10 mg/100 mL. From the results of the lab work, you know that his medication dose

   a. needs to be increased.

   b. needs to be decreased.

   c. needs to be discontinued.

   d. is adequate.

3. Mrs. P. is taking thyroid preparations for hypothyroidism. Which of the following would be indicative of an improvement in her condition?

   a. Normoactive reflexes

   b. Weight gain

   c. Long menstrual periods

   d. Decreased appetite

4. Which of the following diagnoses is appropriate for someone with hypothyroidism?

   a. Altered bowel elimination: diarrhea

   b. Altered nutrition: less than body requirements

   c. Risk for infection

   d. Decreased cardiac output

5. Children who are receiving thyroid replacement should have which of the following parameters monitored regularly?

   a. Urine specific gravity

   b. Muscle mass

   c. Intellectual development

   d. Pulmonary function

6. Which of the following drugs, when administered concurrently with thyroid hormones, increases their effects?

   a. Antidepressants

   b. Beta-adrenergic blockers

   c. Oral contraceptives

   d. Antihypertensives

7. Persons with hypothyroidism are especially sensitive to opioids and sedatives and should be observed for which of the following when they are administered?

   a. Confusion

   b. Tachycardia

   c. Respiratory depression

   d. Hypertension

8. Persons taking propylthiouracil (Propacil) should be instructed about the adverse effects of the medication, which includes

   a. tachycardia.

   b. blood dyscrasias.

   c. edema of the eyelids.

   d. hypertension.

9. Ms. G., a 22-year-old, is to be started on a thyroid preparation. Which of the following questions is important to ask her before initiating treatment?

   a. "Have you ever had elevated blood pressure?"

   b. "Are you presently using birth control pills?"

   c. "Do you take aspirin on a regular basis?"

   d. "Do you have a history of respiratory problems?"

10. When assessing a client on thyroid replacement for hypothyroidism, you should monitor the client for

    a. hypertension.

    b. insomnia.

    c. bradycardia.

    d. weight gain.

■ Critical Thinking Case Study

Mrs. G., a 21-year-old woman, has lost 10 lb since she was seen by her physician 1 year ago. She complains of headaches, insomnia, excessive perspiration, and palpitations. Her vital signs are BP 100/60, pulse 120, respirations 16. Her physician diagnoses her with hyperthyroidism and starts her on propylthiouracil (Propacil) and propranolol (Inderal).

1. Identify which of Mrs. G.'s signs and symptoms are attributable to hyperthyroidism.

2. Explain to Mrs. G. why her physician ordered propranolol (Inderal) and propylthiouracil (Propacil), how long she will need to take the medications, and when she can expect to see therapeutic effects from the medications.

3. Describe the instructions that you will give Mrs. G. regarding the adverse effects of the medications she is taking.

Two years after her initial treatment, Mrs. G. returns to the physician. She has gained 20 lb and complains of being tired. The physician orders thyroid function studies and finds the results to be below the normal range. He starts Mrs. G. on 0.125 mg of Synthroid.

4. Identify why hypothyroidism must be treated.

5. Describe the instructions you will give Mrs. G. regarding Synthroid.

CHAPTER 26

Hormones That Regulate Calcium and Bone Metabolism

■ Fill in the Blanks

Complete the following sentences.

1. Calcium and phosphorus metabolism is regulated by _____ and _____, as well as vitamin D.

2. Generally, when serum calcium levels go _____, serum phosphate levels go _____.

3. When calcium levels are low, the effect of parathyroid hormone on the following tissues is

   a. Bone: _____.

   b. Intestine: _____.

   c. Kidneys: _____.

4. Calcitonin _____ serum calcium levels by decreasing movement of calcium from _____ to _____. It has little effect on _____ calcium metabolism.

5. Vitamin D is obtained from _____ and _____. The main action of vitamin D is to raise _____ by _____ intestinal absorption of dietary calcium and _____.

6. Deficiency of vitamin D causes inadequate absorption of _____ and _____.

7. Low serum calcium levels produce inadequate mineralization of the bone, which causes _____.

8. Calcium is important in the regulation of

   a. _____.
   b. _____.
   c. _____.
   d. _____.
   e. _____.
   f. _____.
   g. _____.
   h. _____.

9. The adult daily calcium requirement is _____.

10. Sources of calcium include _____, _____, _____, _____, _____, and _____.

11. Phosphorus is important because it

    a. _____.
    b. _____.
    c. _____.
    d. _____.
    e. _____.

12. Other than milk products, good sources of phosphorus include _____, _____, _____, _____, and _____.

13. Clinical manifestations of hypocalcemia are characterized by increased _____, which may progress to _____.

14. Severe hypocalcemia may cause _____ and _____.

15. Hypercalcemia is caused by _____, _____, _____, _____, _____, _____, and _____; ingestion of _____, _____, or _____, and _____ in hospitalized clients.

16. Persons using the following drugs are at high risk for developing osteoporosis: _____, _____, and _____.

17. Calcitonin-salmon (Calcimar) _____ serum calcium levels.

18. Furosemide (_____) _____ calcium excretion in urine by preventing its reabsorption in renal tubules.

19. Hypercalcemia can lead to calcium deposits in the kidneys, which may lead to _____ and _____.

20. Plicamycin (Mithracin) lowers serum calcium by _____.

21. Normal saline inhibits _____.

22. For clients experiencing hypercalcemia, fluids should be increased to _____ mL/day.

■ True or False

1. _____ Women over 50 can benefit from calcium and vitamin D supplements.

2. _____ Administration of laxatives can cause hypercalcemia.

3. _____ If calcium is given to a digitalized client, the risk of digitalis toxicity increases.

4. _____ Persons receiving anticonvulsant therapy are likely to develop hypercalcemia.

5. _____ Oral calcium preparations should not be administered with tetracycline because they affect its absorption.

■ Review Questions

1. Administration of which of the following will cause decreased serum calcium levels?
   a. Prednisone (Deltasone)
   b. Calcitriol (Rocaltrol)
   c. Cholecalciferol (Delta-D)
   d. Dihydrotachysterol (Hytakerol)

2. Which of the following electrolyte imbalances will lower serum calcium levels?
   a. Hyperphosphatemia
   b. High serum albumin levels
   c. Low serum sodium levels
   d. Hypokalemia

3. When Mrs. J. is admitted to the hospital, a low serum calcium level is discovered. Which of the following might you expect Mrs. J. to complain of?
   a. Headache and dizziness
   b. Drowsiness
   c. Muscle flaccidity
   d. Numbness and tingling in lips and hands

4. Which statement would lead you to believe that your client understands the teaching that you have done regarding calcium supplements?
   a. "I will take the medication 30 minutes before meals or at bedtime."
   b. "I will take the calcium with antacids to prevent nausea."
   c. "I will contact my physician immediately if I become constipated."
   d. "I must limit my intake of foods high in vitamin K."

5. Your client is admitted with respiratory alkalosis. Which electrolyte imbalance should you assess for?
   a. Hypercalcemia
   b. Hypocalcemia
   c. Hypophosphatemia
   d. Hyperkalemia

6. Mrs. C. has a low serum calcium level. Which of the following foods should you recommend?
   a. Red meat
   b. Whole grains
   c. Dark green leafy vegetables
   d. Citrus fruits

7. Mrs. H. is experiencing acute hypercalcemia. The treatment of choice is

 a. phosphate salts (Neutra-Phos) and a high fruit intake.

 b. etidronate (Didronel) and D$_5$W.

 c. calcitonin-salmon (Calcimar) and lactated Ringer's.

 d. furosemide (Lasix) and normal saline.

8. Mrs. D. is admitted with a serum calcium level of 12.5 mg/dL. You know that this is

 a. below the therapeutic range.

 b. within the therapeutic range.

 c. above the therapeutic range.

 d. extremely high.

9. Mrs. B., who is taking calcium, should avoid concurrent use of the following because it decreases the effects of calcium:

 a. alcohol.

 b. vitamin D.

 c. bran.

 d. laxatives.

10. Ms. J. is taking calcium supplements, and her physician starts her on tetracycline. Which of the following instructions should she receive?

 a. "Take these medications with meals."

 b. "Take both medications on an empty stomach."

 c. "Take tetracycline an hour before meals and calcium with meals."

 d. "Take medications 3 hours apart."

■ Critical Thinking Case Study

J.C. is admitted to your unit in acute renal failure with the following lab values: creatinine 3.8, calcium 12.8 mg/100 mL, potassium 6.8. The physician orders furosemide (Lasix) 40 mg IV, hydrocortisone (Solu-Cortef) 40 mg IV, and 1000 mL 0.9% NaCl to run at 50 mL/hr. (The learner will need additional sources to answer the questions.)

1. Identify what you will be assessing for when J.C. is admitted.

2. Discuss the rationale for the treatment plan.

A dual lumen catheter is inserted and J.C. is dialyzed. When J.C. returns from dialysis, he complains of a headache and nausea.

3. Identify what you will do next.

J.C. is to continue to take furosemide (Lasix) once he returns home.

4. Identify the teaching that you will do with J.C. and his mother to prepare them for discharge.

CHAPTER 27

Antidiabetic Agents

■ Fill in the Blanks

Use the following terms to fill in the blanks.

Increases

Decreases

1. Insulin

   a. _____ storage of glycogen and fatty acids.

   b. _____ the breakdown of glucose.

   c. _____ protein breakdown.

   d. _____ protein and glycogen synthesis.

   e. _____ production of glycerol and fatty acids.

   f. _____ breakdown of fats.

   g. _____ blood glucose levels.

■ Matching Exercise

TERMS AND CONCEPTS

Match the concept with the term for it.

1. _____ A type of hyperglycemia that occurs following an insulin-induced hypoglycemia reaction.

2. _____ Changes in fatty subcutaneous tissue occurring from frequent injections.

3. _____ Persons requiring large doses of insulin, possibly due to the development of antibodies.

4. _____ Symptoms include tachycardia, blurred vision, weakness, fatigue, and sweating.

5. _____ This drug increases the effects of oral agents.

6. _____ This drug raises blood glucose levels and antagonizes the effects of insulin.

7. _____ The normal range for blood glucose levels.

8. _____ Regular insulin peaks.

9. _____ This test reflects the average blood sugar for 2–3 months.

10. _____ A common complication that persons with diabetes experience.

A. Hyperglycemia

B. MAO inhibitors

C. Somogyi effect

D. Lipodystrophy

E. Allopurinol (Zyloprim)

F. Insulin resistance

G. 80–120 mg/100 mL

H. Hypoglycemia

I. Oral contraceptives

J. 60–100 mg/100 mL

K. 2–3 hours

L. 4–6 hours

M. Glycosylated hemoglobin

N. Urinary tract infections

■ Crossword Puzzle

ACROSS

5. A second-generation sulfonylurea, which may cause hypoglycemia in persons with liver disease.

7. Used to treat type 1 diabetes mellitus.

8. This oral antidiabetic drug has been approved for use with insulin.

10. These drugs taken with insulin can increase the chance of hypoglycemia.

12. This reaction to insulin includes tachycardia, hunger, muscle tremors, and blurred vision.

DOWN

1. This type of insulin is preferred for most insulin-dependent diabetic clients.

2. Isotonic IV fluids are an important part of treating diabetic _____.

3. An insulin sensitizer.

4. A first-generation sulfonylurea.

6. Failing to change insulin injection sites can lead to this.

9. Lack of insulin leads to high blood _____ levels.

■ True or False

1. _____ Early symptoms of diabetic ketoacidosis include blurred vision, anorexia, nausea, vomiting, thirst, and polyuria.

2. _____ Insulin can be stored at room temperature.

3. _____ Clients with type 2 diabetes require only oral agents to control their diabetes mellitus.

4. _____ Oral agents are contraindicated during pregnancy.

5. _____ Once insulin has been started, the person will remain on the medication for the rest of his or her life.

6. _____ Symptoms of hypoglycemia include excessive thirst, hunger, and increased urine output.

7. _____ Salicylates taken with antidiabetic drugs increase the likelihood of hypoglycemia.

8. _____ Persons taking adrenocorticosteroids and thiazide diuretics will require less insulin.

9. _____ Insulin is necessary for normal growth and development in children.

10. _____ When treating hypoglycemia, the primary goal is to restore the brain's supply of glucose.

11. _____ A honeymoon period, characterized by recovery of islet function and temporary production of insulin, may occur after diabetes is first diagnosed and treated.

12. _____ Once hypoglycemia is relieved, the client should consume foods high in fat to replace glycogen stores and prevent secondary hypoglycemia.

13. _____ A client with diabetes may take both oral agents and insulin.

■ Review Questions

1. Mr. J. is receiving short- and intermediate-acting insulin in the morning. The most likely time of occurrence for hypoglycemic reactions is
   a. 10 AM and 4 PM
   b. 8 AM and 4 PM
   c. 11 AM and 6 PM
   d. 11 AM and 3 PM

2. Which of the following instructions should be given to a person taking insulin?
   a. "Draw up NPH insulin first, then regular insulin."
   b. "Inject insulin at a 45-degree angle in the subcutaneous tissue."
   c. "Shake the NPH insulin thoroughly before administering it."
   d. "Rotate injection sites; use upper back and buttocks as well as arms, thighs, and abdomen."

3. Which of the following statements by your client leads you to believe that he needs additional teaching about diabetes?
   a. "I will weigh myself weekly and try to maintain my present weight."
   b. "After I begin feeling shaky, I have about 15 minutes before my blood sugar drops dangerously low."
   c. "I will test my blood sugar before and after I exercise."
   d. "I will avoid alcohol and concentrated sweets."

4. Prolonged hypoglycemia resulting from the administration of insulin can result in
   a. kidney damage.
   b. brain damage.
   c. hypoxia.
   d. hypotension.

5. A type 2 non–insulin-dependent diabetic client may require insulin as a result of all of the following except:
   a. surgery.
   b. pregnancy.
   c. infection.
   d. weight loss.

6. Mrs. J. is a type 2 diabetic client who has recently been placed on insulin. Which of the following statements by Mrs. J. leads you to believe that she has understood the teaching that you have done?
   a. "I must take shots now because the oral insulin is no longer effective."
   b. "I know I must keep insulin refrigerated."
   c. "Human insulin is derived from human pancreas."
   d. "I will make sure the insulin I inject is not cold."

7. Administration of which of the following drugs can result in drug-induced diabetes mellitus?
   a. Antidiabetic agents
   b. Beta-adrenergic blockers
   c. Corticosteroids
   d. Loop diuretics

8. Mr. J.'s blood glucose comes back as 130 mg/100 mL. This value is
   a. below the normal range.
   b. within the normal range.
   c. above the normal range.
   d. extremely high.

9. When teaching Mr. J. about the signs and symptoms of hyperglycemia, you tell him he may experience
   a. sweating.
   b. polyuria.
   c. weakness.
   d. dizziness.

10. Which of the following statements is false?
    a. Weight loss will decrease insulin needs in diabetic clients.
    b. Oral agents and insulin cannot be used together.
    c. Regular insulin is the only type of insulin that may be given intravenously.
    d. Insulin pumps use Humalog insulin.

■ Critical Thinking Case Study

Mrs. J. is newly diagnosed with type 1 diabetes mellitus. She takes 3 U Regular Humulin Insulin and 14 U NPH Humulin Insulin in the morning, and 6 U Regular and 10 U NPH before dinner. She experiences frequent hypoglycemia reactions during the next month. One month after starting the regimen, she is brought to the emergency room with lethargy, confusion, and tachycardia. The physician diagnoses her with diabetic ketoacidosis and starts an intravenous solution of normal saline. When you interview Mrs. J., you discover that she had the flu and has been vomiting.

1. Identify the information you will share with Mrs. J. and her husband about diet and lifestyle changes to help her control her diabetes.

Mrs. J. calls her physician because she is having frequent hypoglycemia reactions in the middle of the night.

2. Identify what information you will discuss with Mrs. J. that will help her manage her hypoglycemia.

Mr. J. calls the emergency room and states that his wife is unresponsive and asks you what to do.

3. Discuss your response to Mr. J.

Mrs. J.'s physician changes her insulin to 3 U Regular Insulin and 14 U NPH in the morning, 6 U Regular Insulin at dinnertime, and 10 U of NPH at h.s.

4. Discuss why these changes were made.

CHAPTER 28

Estrogen, Progestins, and Oral Contraceptives

■ True or False

1. _____ The use of estrogen may aggravate gall-bladder disease.

2. _____ Estrogen decreases HDL and increases LDL.

3. _____ Progesterone stimulates milk production.

4. _____ Estrogen has been used to prevent ostero-porosis.

5. _____ During pregnancy the placenta produces large amounts of estrogen.

6. _____ Estrogen decreases vascularity in skin.

7. _____ Progesterone decreases gastrointestinal motility.

8. _____ Women with diabetes mellitus may not use birth control pills.

9. _____ Ovral is prescribed as a postcoital contra-ceptive.

10. _____ Estrogen and progestins should be taken on an empty stomach.

11. _____ Estrogen enhances blood coagulation.

12. _____ Common adverse effects of supplemental estrogen include bleeding and weight gain.

13. _____ Acne is an adverse effect of taking birth control pills.

14. _____ Birth control pills may only be taken for 5 years.

15. _____ Progestins reduce the risk of endometrial cancer in women.

■ Fill in the Blanks

Complete the following sentence.

1. Estrogen is administered in postmenopausal women to prevent

   a. _____.

   b. _____.

   c. _____.

   d. _____.

■ Name That Drug

1. _____ Administered via patch, worn 3 consecutive weeks a month.

2. _____ Used topically for atrophic or senile vaginitis.

3. _____ Administered twice a day for 5 days for postcoital contraception.

4. _____ Can be administered intra-venously for dysfunctional uterine bleeding.

5. _____ Progestin used to treat uter-ine adenocarcinoma.

6. _____ Given intramuscularly in doses of 1.5–2 mg once a month to treat female hypogonadism.

7. _____ A subdermal contraceptive.

8. _____ Used for endometrial cancer, administered intramuscularly weekly until improvement, then monthly.

9. _____ Used to treat breast cancer.

10. _____ This drug is used to prevent osteoporosis in postmenopausal women.

11. _____ This drug decreases the effects of oral anticoagulants, insulin, oral antidiabetic agents, and antihypertensive drugs.

12. _____ This drug is used to treat ovarian failure.

13. _____ This drug is a progestin used to treat endometriosis.

14. _____ An oral contraceptive that contains no estrogen.

15. _____ If this aminoglycoside is administered with oral contraceptives, it will decrease their effectiveness.

■ Review Questions

1. Persons using birth control pills need to be assessed regularly for
   a. increased intraocular pressure.
   b. decreased urinary output.
   c. bradycardia.
   d. hypertension.

2. Mr. B., a 76-year-old man, is started on estrogen for metastatic prostatic cancer. Which of the following statements by Mr. B. leads you to believe he has understood the teaching that you have done?
   a. "I will take the medication on an empty stomach."
   b. "I may experience impotence, which will subside when the drug is stopped."
   c. "If my breasts become enlarged, I will apply ice to them."
   d. "I will take this medication for the rest of my life."

3. Mrs. K. is a 34-year-old mother of two with a history of diabetes and cancer of the breast. She is on a low-residue diet for colitis. Which of the factors in Mrs. K.'s history would contraindicate the use of birth control pills?
   a. Cancer of the breast
   b. Age
   c. Diabetes
   d. Colitis

4. Estropipate (Ogen) is administered to women for
   a. atrophic vaginitis.
   b. dysfunctional uterine bleeding.
   c. osteoporosis.
   d. uterine cancer.

5. Which of the following medications is administered for treatment of breast cancer?
   a. Estropipate (Ogen)
   b. Medroxyprogesterone acetate (Depo-Provera)
   c. Estradiol cypionate (Depo-Estradiol)
   d. Megestrol acetate (Megace)

6. Which of the following statements indicates that your client needs additional teaching about birth control pills?
   a. "I will monitor my weight and have my blood pressure checked monthly."
   b. "I may gain weight while I am taking these pills."
   c. "I will elevate my legs and take aspirin if I experience leg pain."
   d. "I know nausea is common, but it should subside in a few weeks."

7. The following instructions should be included before estrone (Theelin) is started for dysfunctional uterine bleeding. "You will take the medication…"
   a. "daily until the bleeding is controlled, followed by progestin for 1 week."
   b. "twice a day until the bleeding subsides, followed by a week of prophylactic therapy."
   c. "three times a day until the bleeding stops."
   d. "intramuscularly daily until the bleeding stops, followed by 2 weeks of the oral preparation."

8. Which of the following statements by Mrs. G. leads you to believe that she has a good understanding of how to treat postpartum breast engorgement?
   a. "I will take the Tylenol twice a day for 2 weeks."
   b. "I will take the aspirin q6h for six doses."
   c. "I should decrease my fluid intake."
   d. "If I experience swelling, I should go to the emergency room immediately."

9. Which of the following medications, when administered concurrently with oral contraceptives, will decrease their effect?

   a. Antimicrobials

   b. Antihypertensives

   c. Anticoagulants

   d. Diabetic agents

10. Ms. G. has female hypogonadism and is being treated with estrogen. Which of the following statements leads you to believe that she has a good understanding about the medication?

    a. "I need to eat foods high in fiber."

    b. "I will weigh myself daily and call the doctor if I lose weight."

    c. "I will take the medication for the rest of my life."

    d. "I may experience breast enlargement or growth of hair in the pubic area."

■ Critical Thinking Case Study

Ms. G. has come to the gynecologist requesting birth control pills.

1. Identify what factors would contraindicate the use of birth control pills and why.

2. Identify the assessments that should be done before birth control is started.

Ms. G. calls you, after taking birth control pills for 2 months, stating that she has severe acne and has gained 5 pounds.

3. Identify your response to Ms. G.

CHAPTER 29

Androgens and Anabolic Steroids

■ Circle the Correct Answer

1. There will be a(an) increase/decrease in skin thickness when androgens or anabolic steroids are administered.

2. With the administration of androgens or anabolic steroids, protein anabolism increases/decreases and protein catabolism increases/decreases.

3. When anabolic steroids are administered, there is a(an) increased/decreased secretion of FSH.

4. Administration of testosterone to women increases/decreases the lining of the uterus.

5. Persons taking androgens or anabolic steroids will notice a(an) increase/decrease in muscle mass.

6. When androgens are administered to young children, the result will be a significant increase/decrease in growth.

7. Androgens increase/decrease the development of female sexual characteristics.

8. When androgens or anabolic steroids are administered, there will be a(an) increase/decrease in body weight.

9. Large amounts of anabolic steroids ingested by adult males can cause a(an) increased/decreased sperm count.

10. Administration of androgens or anabolic steroids results in a(an) increase/decrease in sodium and water retention.

11. Administration of anabolic steroids increases/decreases the risk of developing prostatic cancer.

12. Testosterone causes an increase or decrease in bone growth.

13. Persons taking anabolic steroids have documented a(an) increase/decrease in body hair.

14. Ingestion of anabolic steroids results in increased/decreased lipid levels.

15. Androgens increase/decrease the rate of epiphyseal closure in children.

16. Barbiturates administered concurrently with androgens will increase/decrease the effects of androgens.

17. Androgens increase/decrease the effect of insulin.

18. Androgens can increase/decrease blood pressure in the elderly.

19. Androgens can increase/decrease the size of the prostate gland.

20. An effect of the administration of anabolic steroids is increased/decreased acne.

21. Athletes using anabolic steriods will experience an increase/decrease in aggression.

■ Crossword Puzzle

ACROSS

2. This drug's dosage may need to be decreased during androgen treatment.

3. One dangerous side effect of anabolic steroid use is an _____ imbalance.

5. Androgen therapy in children can lead to premature _____ closure.

6. Used for treatment of hypogonadism.

7. Administration of anabolic steriods to males can result in _____.

8. The trade name for nandrolone.

9. Use of anabolic steriods can result in _____.

DOWN

1. Used to treat endometriosis and fibrocystic breast disease.

3. This type of androgen may be given orally.

4. Produced in the human body by Leydig's cells.

■ Review Questions

1. Which of the following medications, if administered concurrently with anabolic steroids, will decrease their effects?
   a. Calcium channel blockers
   b. Barbiturates
   c. Thiazide diuretics
   d. Anticholinergic drugs

2. Persons taking anabolic steroids may experience which of the following beneficial effects?
   a. Increased muscle mass
   b. Decreased appetite
   c. Increased secretion of FSH and LH
   d. Decreased serum sodium levels

3. Physical changes that occur with the use of anabolic steroids in women include
   a. thinning of skin.
   b. increased menstrual flow.
   c. increased distribution of hair on body.
   d. increased endurance.

4. When androgens are administered to older adult males, which of the following can result?
   a. Gynecomastia
   b. Rapid bone growth
   c. Loss of pubic hair
   d. Prostatic enlargement

5. When androgens are administered, an expected outcome is increased
   a. appetite.
   b. serum albumin levels.
   c. serum potassium level.
   d. sperm count.

6. Mrs. A. is receiving danazol (Danocrine) for fibrocystic breast disease. Which of the following should she have checked regularly?
   a. Renal function
   b. Pulse rate
   c. Hematocrit
   d. Liver function

7. Androgens can cause
   a. hyperkalemia.
   b. osteoporosis.
   c. hypotension.
   d. sodium and water retention.

8. Mrs. H. is receiving androgens. An adverse reaction resulting from the administration of this medication that the nurse needs to assess for is
   a. hypocalcemia.
   b. jaundice.
   c. skin rash.
   d. oliguria.

9. Androgens can potentiate the effect of oral antidiabetic agents. The dose of the oral antidiabetic drugs may need to be
   a. decreased.
   b. increased.
   c. stopped.
   d. changed to insulin.

10. Testosterone enanthate (Delatestryl) is ordered for B.J., age 11, who is experiencing hypogonadism. Which of the following statements by B.J. leads you to believe that he has understood the teaching that you have done regarding the medication?
   a. "I may experience visual changes as a result of taking this drug."
   b. "I will need to see the doctor every 6 months for x-rays."
   c. "If I experience acne, the drug will need to be stopped."
   d. "I can expect to lose weight as a result of taking this drug."

■ Critical Thinking Case Study

You are the school nurse at East Side High School. The wrestling coach asks you to give a presentation on anabolic steroids.

1. Develop a presentation that would convince teenage boys not to use anabolic steroids.

2. Identify ways the school nurse can monitor the health of high school athletes and possibly detect the use of steroids.

CHAPTER 30

Nutritional Support Products and Drugs for Obesity

■ Fill in the Blanks

Place a P for protein, a C for carbohydrate, a W for water, or an F for fat next to each body function. More than one nutrient may be listed for each body function.

1. _____ Furnishes amino acids.

2. _____ Necessary for excretion of metabolic waste.

3. _____ Anatomic component of all cells.

4. _____ Sources of energy for cellular metabolism.

5. _____ Promotes cellular metabolism.

■ True or False

1. _____ An increased hematocrit is indicative of fluid volume excess.

2. _____ Phenylpropanolamine has been associated with psychosis.

3. _____ Undernutrition can cause tachycardia and hypertension.

4. _____ Enteral nutrition cannot be used if the client has an ileus.

5. _____ Persons who are obese are more susceptible to developing an infection than undernourished persons.

6. _____ Some tube feedings are better tolerated if they are diluted initially.

7. _____ Intermittent feedings are preferable because diarrhea and gastric distention are decreased.

8. _____ A nasogastric tube will prevent the complication of aspiration.

9. _____ Pancreatic enzymes should be administered with food.

10. _____ Cold tube feedings are better tolerated than those at room temperature.

11. _____ Persons with MODS need large amounts of fat.

12. _____ Fat emulsion cannot be mixed with TPN solution.

■ Matching Exercise

Match the formula or elemental diet with the population for which it is intended.

1. _____ Portagen

2. _____ Pulmocare

3. _____ Nutramigen

4. _____ NephrAmine

5. _____ Isomil

6. _____ Pregestimil

7. _____ Vivonex

8. _____ Lofenalac

9. _____ TraumaCal

10. _____ Nepro

11. _____ HepatAmine

12. _____ Liposyn

A. Infants with malabsorption syndromes.

B. Persons with chronic obstructive pulmonary disease.

C. Persons with fat and malabsorption problems.

D. Persons with GI disorders, because it requires no digestion and leaves no fecal residue.

E. Persons allergic to milk.

F. Children who are allergic to ordinary proteins.

G. Amino acid solution for persons with renal failure.

H. Patients on dialysis use this formula.

I. Burn injury victims.

J. Children with phenylketonuria.

K. Persons with hepatic encephalopathy and coma use this.

L. A component of TPN.

■ Fill in the Blanks

Complete the following sentences.

1. A frequently used dextrose solution is _____ in _____ or _____.

2. For total parenteral nutrition, _____ and _____ glucose solutions are used. They are _____, so they must be given through a central line.

3. Five hundred milliliters of a 10% fat emulsion provides _____ calories.

4. When a person is receiving tube feedings, additional _____ is necessary between feedings.

5. Most tube feedings are _____ and will therefore _____ a fluid volume deficit if water is not administered with them.

6. TPN or hyperalimentation contains _____ and _____.

7. Fat emulsions provide _____ and can be administered _____ or _____.

8. Before administering a tube feeding, the nurse should check _____.

9. The maximum amount of a tube feeding, including water, that should be administered at any one time is _____.

10. Clients receiving 2000 mL/day of tube feeding daily should receive _____ mL of water.

■ Review Questions

1. 500 mL of a 10% fat emulsion provides
   a. 170 calories.
   b. 220 calories.
   c. 300 calories.
   d. 550 calories.

2. 1000 mL of $D_{10}W$ provides
   a. 340 calories.
   b. 480 calories.
   c. 550 calories.
   d. 1000 calories.

3. Which of the following, if administered concurrently with anorexiants, will decrease their effect?
   a. Sodium bicarbonate
   b. Tricyclic antidepressants
   c. Vitamin C
   d. Epinephrine

4. Which of the following liquid formulas is the most appropriate for a baby who has diarrhea or a malabsorption syndrome?
   a. Portagen
   b. Pediasure
   c. Pregestimil
   d. Lofenalac

5. Persons receiving anorexiant drugs that contain phenylpropanolamine should be instructed about the adverse effects, which include
   a. hepatotoxicity.
   b. weakness, dizziness, and blurred vision.
   c. increased blood pressure.
   d. nausea, vomiting, and diarrhea.

6. Persons receiving TPN (total parenteral nutrition) should be observed for
   a. fluid deficit and metabolic acidosis.
   b. increased urinary output.
   c. elevated blood glucose levels.
   d. lower serum sodium levels.

7. A physician has ordered Polycose for M.J., a burn victim, because it
   a. is a high-protein substance, which M.J. needs right now.
   b. supplies a concentrated source of calories, protein, and electrolytes.
   c. is an additive that is mixed with food or beverages to increase the caloric intake.
   d. is an oral supplement that will increase M.J.'s protein, vitamin, and mineral intake.

8. Mr. P. is receiving a fat emulsion and begins complaining of dyspnea and chest pain. Identify what your first nursing action should be.
   a. Slow down the rate of the infusion.
   b. Check Mr. P.'s vital signs.
   c. Contact Mr. P.'s physician.
   d. Stop the fat emulsion infusion.

9. Your client, who has a 10-year history of chronic renal failure, is to receive Amin Aid for his supplemental feedings because
   a. it supplies amino acids, carbohydrates, and a few electrolytes.
   b. its metabolism produces less carbon dioxide.
   c. it is high in nitrogen and high in carbohydrates.
   d. it requires no digestion and leaves no fecal residue.

10. Mrs. J., who is admitted with severe dehydration, will have a(n)
    a. elevated hematocrit.
    b. low serum sodium.
    c. protein deficit.
    d. low serum potassium.

■ Critical Thinking Case Study

Mr. J. is a 76-year-old man with a 10-year history of COPD. His most recent hospital admission is for a CVA. He is unresponsive and has a large pressure sore on his coccyx. A nasogastric tube is inserted, and he is to receive 80 mL of Pulmocare and 40 mL of water per hour in continuous feedings.

1. Identify why Pulmocare was chosen for the supplemental feeding for Mr. J.

2. Identify the nursing assessment that you will do for Mr. J.

3. Discuss the advantages and disadvantages of TPN and parenteral feedings, and identify why Mr. J. was started on tube feeding instead of TPN.

4. Identify potential problems that a client with a tube feeding can experience and how these problems can be avoided.

Mr. J. experiences diarrhea four times during your shift.

5. Identify your nursing actions.

CHAPTER 31

Vitamins

■ Matching Exercise

TERMS AND CONCEPTS

Match the concept with the term for it.

1. _____ Required for normal vision.

2. _____ Found in cereals, green vegetables, egg yolk, and vegetable oils.

3. _____ Essential for normal clotting.

4. _____ Essential in fat and carbohydrate metabolism.

5. _____ Necessary for the normal development of RBCs and for growth.

6. _____ Found in liver, kidney beans, and green vegetables.

7. _____ Essential for fat synthesis.

8. _____ Necessary for the synthesis of cholesterol.

9. _____ Helps maintain cellular immunity.

10. _____ May function in production of corticosteroids and RBCs and in gluconeogenesis.

11. _____ Found in dried beans, whole grains, and peanuts.

12. _____ Not stored in body to a significant extent; excess excreted in the urine.

13. _____ Fat-soluble vitamin obtained from exposure of skin to sunlight.

A. Folic acid (folate)

B. Niacin (vitamin B_3)

C. Riboflavin (vitamin B_2)

D. Vitamin A

E. Pantothenic acid (vitamin B_5)

F. Vitamin E

G. Thiamine (vitamin B_1)

H. Vitamin K

I. Pyridoxine (vitamin B_6)

J. Biotin

K. Vitamin D

L. Cyanocobalamin (vitamin B_{12})

M. Vitamin C (ascorbic acid)

■ Name That Deficiency/Excess

Specify a vitamin and deficiency or excess for each condition. More than one vitamin may relate to a condition.

1. _____ Causes night blindness.

2. _____ Results in bleeding abnormalities.

3. _____ Symptoms include anorexia, nausea, depression, and muscle pain.

4. _____ Causes convulsions, peripheral neuritis, and mental depression.

5. _____ Can cause renal calculi.

6. _____ Causes Wernicke-Korsakoff syndrome.

7. _____ Neurologic symptoms of this disorder include paresthesia, unsteady gait, and depressed deep tendon reflexes.

8. _____ Can cause scurvy.

9. _____ Causes impaired growth in children.

10. _____ Increases intracranial pressure.

11. _____ May be caused by smoking.

12. _____ Causes eye disorders (burning, itching, photophobia).

13. _____ Causes delusions, hallucinations, and impaired peripheral motor function.

14. _____ Can increase the amounts of oxalate in urine.

15. _____ Causes pernicious anemia.

16. _____ Results from a lack of hydrochloric acid or intrinsic factor in the stomach.

17. _____ Occurs commonly in newborns.

18. _____ Early manifestations include anorexia, vomiting, irritability, and skin changes.

19. _____ Alcoholism is a common cause.

20. _____ Persons using oral contraceptives are at risk for developing this.

■ Review Questions

1. Which of the following is a fat-soluble vitamin that may cause toxicity?
   a. Vitamin A
   b. Vitamin B_6
   c. Vitamin C
   d. Folic acid (Folvite)

2. The adverse effects of administering large amounts of vitamin C include development of
   a. skin rashes.
   b. kidney stones.
   c. constipation.
   d. elevated uric acid levels.

3. A vitamin deficiency commonly found in alcoholics that is treated with vitamin supplementation is
   a. pantothenic acid (vitamin B_5) deficiency.
   b. vitamin A deficiency.
   c. vitamin D deficiency.
   d. thiamine (vitamin B_1) deficiency.

4. An expected outcome of the administration of vitamin B_{12} is
   a. decreased appetite.
   b. increased strength.
   c. decreased joint pain.
   d. improved vision.

5. The antidote for warfarin (Coumadin) is
   a. vitamin A.
   b. vitamin B_{12}.
   c. vitamin E.
   d. vitamin K.

6. Mr. J., a homeless man, is found by the side of the road. He is delusional and having auditory and visual hallucinations. His symptoms may be attributed to a deficiency of which of the following vitamins?
   a. Ascorbic acid (vitamin C)
   b. Riboflavin (vitamin B_1)
   c. Pantothenic acid (vitamin B_5)
   d. Niacin (vitamin B_3)

7. Mrs. H. is experiencing fatigue, anorexia, depression, and irritability. A deficiency of which of these vitamins can cause these symptoms?

   a. Vitamin A

   b. Vitamin B_{12} (cyanocobalamin)

   c. Vitamin C (ascorbic acid)

   d. Vitamin B_1 (thiamine)

8. Which of the following statements by your client leads you to believe she has understood the teaching that you have done regarding vitamin B_{12}?

   a. "The intrinsic factor in my stomach that is required for absorption of vitamin B_{12} is absent, so I must take supplemental B_{12}."

   b. "Long-term use of this drug is associated with peripheral neuropathies."

   c. "Pernicious anemia causes changes in the mucous membrane lining and impairs absorption, so I may have diarrhea once I start this drug."

   d. "I will take this medication for a few months until I feel better."

9. A vitamin administered for treatment of hyperlipidemia is

   a. pyridoxine (vitamin B_6).

   b. pantothenic acid (vitamin B_5).

   c. niacin (vitamin B_3).

   d. riboflavin (vitamin B_2).

10. Before administering vitamin B_{12}, the following test(s) may be performed to determine the presence of pernicious anemia:

   a. hematocrit and hemoglobin.

   b. Schick test.

   c. sweat test.

   d. Schilling test.

■ Critical Thinking Case Study

Mr. B., a severely malnourished 56-year-old man with alcoholism, is admitted to your unit. Mr. B.'s physician orders niacin (vitamin B_3), thiamine (vitamin B_1), and folic acid (folate).

1. Specify the nursing assessments that you will do (including analysis of lab studies) when Mr. J. is admitted.

2. Discuss the rationale for using these medications and why they are administered parenterally.

Two days after admission, Mr. B. states, "I will not take any more shots and that is final."

3. Discuss how you will proceed.

CHAPTER 32

Minerals and Electrolytes

■ Matching Exercise

TERMS AND CONCEPTS

Match the concept with the term for it.

1. _____ Necessary for normal cell growth and synthesis of carbohydrates and proteins.

2. _____ Essential component of hemoglobin.

3. _____ Causes skeletal muscle weakness, respiratory insufficiency, and drowsiness.

4. _____ Causes abdominal distension, constipation, and paralytic ileus.

5. _____ This trace element is found in seafood.

6. _____ Strengthens bones by promoting calcium retention.

7. _____ This trace element is found in brain, heart, liver, kidneys, bone, and muscle.

8. _____ A component of vitamin B_{12} that is required for normal function of all body cells.

9. _____ Symptoms include headache, dizziness, weakness, lethargy, restlessness, confusion, and convulsions.

10. _____ An exchange resin used for the treatment of hyperkalemia.

11. _____ A chelating agent used to remove excess iron.

12. _____ Increases the effectiveness of insulin.

13. _____ Assists in regulating osmotic pressure.

14. _____ Eliminated from the body primarily by the kidneys.

15. _____ Shifts in and out of the red blood cells in exchange for bicarbonate.

16. _____ Good food sources include nuts, cereal, grains, seafood, and green vegetables.

A. Copper
B. Hyponatremia
C. Deferoxamine (Desferal Mesylate)
D. Hypermagnesemia
E. Chromium
F. Iron
G. Zinc
H. Hypokalemia
I. Fluoride
J. Sodium
K. Cobalt
L. Potassium
M. Iodine
N. Magnesium
O. Chloride
P. Sodium polystyrene sulfonate (Kayexalate)

■ Name That Imbalance

Specify the imbalance associated with each condition. More than one imbalance may relate to a condition.

1. _____ Causes peaked T waves, prolonged PR intervals, and prolonged QRS complexes.

2. _____ Signs and symptoms include impaired growth, anorexia, loss of taste and smell, and poor wound healing.

3. _____ Results in increased extracellular volume.

4. _____ Occurs in persons who ingest excessive bicarbonate.

5. _____ Can occur as a result of acidosis.

6. _____ Produces impaired glucose tolerance and impaired growth and reproduction.

7. _____ Causes depressed ST segments and inverted T waves.

8. _____ Menke's syndrome is caused by this.

9. _____ Hypotension is a symptom of this.

10. _____ May result in coma.

11. _____ Hyperaldosteronism and Cushing's disease can cause this.

12. _____ Results in impaired erythropoiesis.

13. _____ Can result in increased BUN and oliguria.

14. _____ Results in skeletal muscle weakness and paralysis.

15. _____ Can result from vomiting and diarrhea.

16. _____ Excessive administration of ammonium chloride can cause this.

17. _____ Muscle spasms and tetany can result from this.

18. _____ Administration of salt substitutes can cause this.

19. _____ Commonly occurs with alcoholism.

20. _____ Causes depressant effects on the neuromuscular system.

■ Review Questions

1. Chromium is a trace element important
   a. for cell growth and synthesis of carbohydrates.
   b. because it increases the effectiveness of insulin.
   c. because it assists in regulating osmotic pressure.
   d. in the formation of red blood cells.

2. Mr. J. is admitted with dehydration. His lab values are Na+ 145 mEq/L, K+ 6 mEq/L, Cl- 95 mEq/L, Mg++ 2.0 mEq/L. Identify the electrolyte imbalance Mr. J. is experiencing.
   a. Hypernatremia
   b. Hyperkalemia
   c. Hypochloremia
   d. Hypomagnesemia

3. The drug of choice for treating hyperkalemia is
   a. sodium bicarbonate.
   b. deferoxamine (Desferal Mesylate).
   c. penicillamine (Cuprimine).
   d. sodium polystyrene sulfonate (Kayexalate).

4. Inadequate ingestion of iron can result in
   a. heart failure.
   b. respiratory failure.
   c. inadequate oxygen supply to cells.
   d. decreased muscle mass.

5. Iodine can be found in
   a. citrus fruits.
   b. seafood.
   c. wheat germ.
   d. red meat.

6. A zinc deficiency can cause
   a. thyroid enlargement.
   b. sensory impairment.
   c. stomatitis.
   d. lymphadenopathy.

7. Mrs. G. is being discharged on a potassium supplement along with a thiazide diuretic. Which of the following statements by Mrs. G. leads you to believe that she has understood the teaching you have done?
   a. "I will check my pulse regularly and contact my physician if there is a significant change."
   b. "I can take the potassium with vitamin C to increase its absorption."
   c. "I will take the medication on an empty stomach an hour before meals."
   d. "I can expect an increase in my appetite in about a week."

8. Symptoms of hypernatremia the nurse needs to observe for, when saline cathartics are administered, include

   a. bradycardia.

   b. diarrhea.

   c. hyperactive reflexes.

   d. headache and dizziness.

9. A person with hyperkalemia should be observed for

   a. muscle rigidity.

   b. hypertension.

   c. dysrhythmias.

   d. seizures.

10. The drug of choice for acute iron intoxication is

    a. sodium bicarbonate.

    b. succimer (Chemet).

    c. penicillamine (Cuprimine).

    d. deferoxamine (Desferal Mesylate).

▪ Critical Thinking Case Study

Mr. B. is seen in the emergency room for chest pain. He has not been feeling well for some time. He has been treated for hypertension for 5 years. His blood pressure is 170/90 and pulse is 110. Laboratory values are BUN 108 mg/dL, creatinine 10 mg/dL, sodium 142 mEq/L, and potassium 7 mEq/L.

1. Identify and prioritize your nursing actions.

The physician diagnoses Mr. B. with renal failure and orders sodium bicarbonate 45 mEq over 15 minutes and 5 mL of 10% calcium gluconate.

2. Identify what you will be assessing for.

Mr. B.'s potassium comes down to 5.9 mEq/L. His physician orders Kayexalate in sorbitol via enema. Mr. B. asks you why the medication must be administered this way.

3. Describe how you will respond to Mr. B.'s inquiry.

CHAPTER **33**

General Characteristics of Antimicrobial Drugs

■ Fill in the Blanks

Complete the following sentences.

1. Three types of organisms that can cause an infection are

   a. _____ .

   b. _____ .

   c. _____ .

2. Normal flora protect the human host by
   _____ .

3. Resistant bacteria can cause _____
   in the original host and spread to
   _____ .

4. Factors that predispose one to infection include

   a. _____ .

   b. _____ .

   c. _____ .

   d. _____ .

   e. _____ .

   f. _____ .

   g. _____ .

   h. _____ .

   i. _____ .

5. A hospital-acquired infection is also referred to as
   a _____ infection.

6. Antimicrobial drugs include _____ ,
   _____ , and _____ .

7. The term _____ refers to killing
   microorganisms.

8. The term _____ refers to inhibition
   of growth of microorganisms.

9. For most acute infections, the average duration of
   treatment with an antibiotic is _____
   days.

10. If your client has renal insufficiency, the dose of
    the antibiotic may need to be _____ .
    The drug dosage is based on the individual's
    _____ clearance.

11. Drugs that may cause nephrotoxicity and ototoxi-
    city include _____ .

12. The following drugs are excreted by the liver and
    their dosage must be reduced with liver impair-
    ment: _____ , _____ ,
    _____ , and _____ .

13. Adverse effects of antibiotics that the nurse should
    observe for include

    a. _____ .

    b. _____ .

    c. _____ .

    d. _____ .

    e. _____ .

    f. _____ .

    g. _____ .

    h. _____ .

14. Common symptoms that can be seen with a super-
    infection are

    a. _____ .

    b. _____ .

    c. _____ .

    d. _____ .

Copyright © 2001. Lippincott Williams & Wilkins.
Study Guide to Accompany Clinical Drug Therapy: Rationales for Nursing Practice, sixth edition, by Gail Ropelewski-Ryan.

109

■ Review Questions

1. If your client has severe liver disease, the dose of antibiotic ordered may need to be
   a. increased.
   b. decreased.
   c. unchanged.
   d. withheld.

2. Persons in hospitals who are immunosuppressed are susceptible to this type of infection.
   a. Nosocomial infection
   b. Communal infection
   c. Sustained infection
   d. Antimicrobial infection

3. For most acute infections, the usual duration of treatment is
   a. 48–72 hours.
   b. 3–5 days.
   c. 7–10 days.
   d. 2–3 weeks.

4. Vaginal *Candida albicans* infection, commonly treated with miconazole (Monistat), is an example of a
   a. gram-positive bacterial infection.
   b. gram-negative bacterial infection.
   c. fungal infection.
   d. viral infection.

5. Which of the following antimicrobials is contraindicated in children under the age of 8?
   a. Penicillin
   b. Cephalosporins
   c. Erythromycin
   d. Tetracyclines

6. Which of the following impairs the body's defense mechanism and makes it more likely that an individual will develop an opportunistic infection?
   a. Therapy with thiazide diuretics
   b. Weight loss
   c. Dehydration
   d. Chronic steroid drug therapy

7. Objective signs of an infection include which of the following?
   a. Lethargy
   b. Nausea
   c. Leukocytosis
   d. Hypertension

8. Prophylactic antibiotics are used with dental procedures for persons with a history of
   a. diabetes mellitus.
   b. renal insufficiency.
   c. asthma.
   d. rheumatic heart disease.

9. Staphylococci organisms normally found in the intestine are referred to as
   a. opportunistic microorganisms.
   b. indigenous flora.
   c. resistant microorganisms.
   d. nosocomial infections.

10. You should assess Mr. J., age 75, for nephrotoxicity and ototoxicity when administering which of the following antimicrobials?
    a. Cefazolin
    b. Clindamycin
    c. Gentamicin
    d. Erythromycin

CHAPTER 34

Beta-Lactam Antibacterials: Penicillins, Cephalosporins, and Others

■ Fill in the Blanks

Complete the following sentences.

1. Penicillins are often effective in treating

   a. _____.

   b. _____.

   c. _____.

   d. _____.

2. Penicillin may be useful in _____,
   _____, or _____
   infections.

3. If an infection is caused by staphylococci that are
   resistant to penicillin G, the following drugs may
   be effective: _____,
   _____, _____, and
   _____.

4. A broad spectrum, semisynthetic penicillin effective against several types of gram-positive and
   gram-negative bacteria is _____.

5. Ampicillin is effective in treating the following
   infections: _____,
   _____, _____, and
   _____.

6. Unasyn is a combination of _____
   and _____.

7. Four penicillins used to treat *Pseudomonas* are
   _____, _____,
   _____, and _____.

8. For pseudomonal infections, a penicillin is used
   concomitantly with a(an) _____.

9. Cephalosporins act against _____
   and _____ organisms.

10. There are _____,
    _____, _____, and
    _____ generation cephalosporins.

11. Cephalosporins are commonly used for surgical
    prophylaxis and infections of the

    a. _____.

    b. _____.

    c. _____.

    d. _____.

    e. _____.

    f. _____.

12. A newer carbapenem used before causative organ-
    isms are identified is _____
    (_____).

■ Crossword Puzzle

ACROSS

1. A patient with an anaphylactic reaction to _____ may be sensitive to cephalosporins as well.

8. Cephalosporins may aggravate _____ impairment.

9. Third-generation cephalosporins can penetrate into _____ fluid and aid meningeal infections.

10. Generic name for Ancef.

11. Contains amoxicillin and potassium clavulanate.

DOWN

2. The first third-generation cephalosporin approved for once daily dosage.

3. First-generation cephalosporins are often used to prevent infections after _____ surgery.

4. A penicillin that is effective against *Pseudomonas* organisms.

5. These drugs decrease the effects of cephalosporins.

6. This drug is excreted in bile, and its half-life is prolonged in hepatic failure.

7. The first oral cephalosporin, still extensively used.

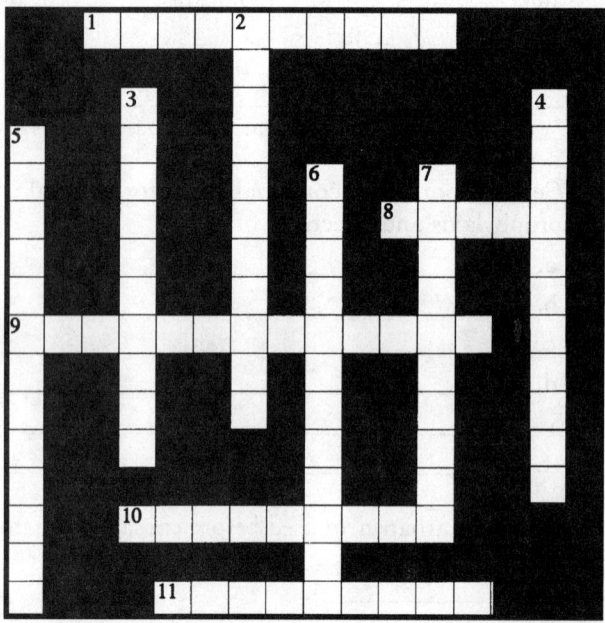

■ Review Questions

1. A penicillin used to treat staphylococcal infections that are resistant to penicillin G is
   a. bacampicillin (Spectrobid).
   b. amoxicillin (Amoxil).
   c. nafcillin (Unipen).
   d. carbenicillin (Geopen).

2. Your client weighs 132 lb and is to receive four doses of Unipen. The total daily dose is 50 mg/kg/day. How much will your client receive per dose?
   a. 500 mg
   b. 750 mg
   c. 2000 mg
   d. 3000 mg

3. After receiving penicillin for 5 days, Mrs. A. complains of soreness in her mouth, diarrhea, and vaginal itching, which may be signs of
   a. anaphylactic reactions to the drug.
   b. spread of her infection.
   c. ineffectiveness of drug therapy.
   d. superimposed infection.

4. When probenecid is administered with penicillin, which of the following results?
   a. Hypersensitivity is common.
   b. Glucosuria
   c. Drug action is decreased.
   d. Drug action is increased.

5. A severe adverse reaction that someone might develop after the administration of a cephalosporin is
   a. hypertension.
   b. pseudomembranous colitis.
   c. diabetes mellitus.
   d. gingivitis.

6. Cefuroxime is used for surgical prophylaxis. When is the best time to administer the medication?
   a. 12 hours before surgery
   b. 2 hours before surgery
   c. 30–60 minutes before surgery
   d. During surgery

7. When administering large doses of ticarcillin (Ticar) IV, the nurse needs to observe for

   a. tachycardia.

   b. jaundice.

   c. bleeding.

   d. hypertension.

8. Which of the following drugs, when administered with cephalosporins, will decrease the therapeutic effects?

   a. Furosemide (Lasix)

   b. Probenecid (Benemid)

   c. Aminoglycoside

   d. Tetracycline

9. Which of the following would be indicative of a cephalosporin allergy and should be reported to the physician?

   a. Nausea, vomiting, and diarrhea

   b. Flushing and swelling of the head and neck

   c. Nasal congestion and itching

   d. Skin rash, drug fever, and eosinophilia

10. Which of the following instructions should be given to Mr. P., who is to be discharged on oral cephalosporins?

   a. "If you see blood, pus, or mucus in your stool, contact the doctor immediately."

   b. "Take the medication on an empty stomach to increase its absorption."

   c. "Do not use antacids while you are taking this medication."

   d. "If your urinary output decreases, cut the dose of the medication in half."

■ Critical Thinking Case Study

Mr. B., a type 1 diabetic client, is admitted to the hospital with severe dehydration. He has recently returned from a trip and has had diarrhea since he returned home. His stool culture reveals *Shigella* organisms, and he is started on ampicillin and sulbactam (Unasyn) IV.

1. Explain why this drug was chosen for Mr. B.

2. Explain the rationale for the route of administration.

The following morning, you enter Mr. B.'s room and find that Mr. B. has a dull, red rash on his face and chest.

3. Identify and prioritize your nursing actions.

CHAPTER 35

Aminoglycosides and Fluoroquinolones

■ Fill in the Blanks

Complete the following sentences.

1. Aminoglycosides are used to treat infections caused by _____ microorganisms.

2. Quinolones are commonly used to treat _____ infections.

3. Aminoglycosides are used intravenously to treat _____ and _____ infections.

4. Streptomycin is used for tuberculosis that is _____.

5. Aminoglycosides are also used orally to suppress _____, which produce _____.

6. Before administering aminoglycosides, the nurse should
   a. _____.
   b. _____.
   c. analyze medications and assess other drugs that interact with _____.

7. While your client is receiving aminoglycosides, monitor _____ and _____, and force fluids to _____ daily.

8. Aminoglycoside dosages are individualized by _____, _____, _____, and _____.

9. With fluoroquinolones, assess for factors that increase risk of _____, _____ and _____.

10. Fluoroquinolones are contraindicated in
    a. _____.
    b. _____.
    c. _____.

11. Peak levels of aminoglycosides should be obtained _____ minutes after a dose. Both peak and _____ levels are necessary to establish a therapeutic serum level. Trough levels are taken 10–15 minutes before the next dose. For gentamicin and tobramycin, peak levels above _____ µg/mL and trough levels above _____ µg/mL have been associated with nephrotoxicity.

12. The half-life of aminoglycosides is _____ hours with normal renal function.

13. When administering aminoglycosides, avoid concurrent administration with _____.

■ Review Questions

1. Aminoglycosides are used orally to treat
   a. gram-positive infections.
   b. gram-negative infections.
   c. fungal infections.
   d. viral infections.

2. The physician orders gentamicin for a child weighing 88 lb. If the dose range is 6–7.5 mg/kg/day, and the child is to receive the medication t.i.d., how many milligrams should the child receive per dose?
   a. 20 mg
   b. 40 mg
   c. 60 mg
   d. 80 mg

3. Which of the following drugs should be avoided when a person is receiving aminoglycosides?
   a. Furosemide (Lasix)
   b. Prednisone
   c. Aspirin
   d. Propranolol (Inderal)

4. Aminoglycosides can be nephrotoxic. The most effective way of preventing compromised renal function in Mr. T. is to
   a. maintain his pulse above 60.
   b. keep him well hydrated.
   c. provide daily exercise to ensure adequate blood flow to the kidneys.
   d. avoid concurrent administration of aminoglycosides with antacids.

5. An aminoglycoside that is used in hepatic coma to decrease intestinal bacteria is
   a. neomycin.
   b. netilmicin (Netromycin).
   c. streptomycin.
   d. tobramycin (Nebcin).

6. This drug is commonly used with gentamicin (Garamycin) to treat *Pseudomonas* infections.
   a. Piperacillin (Pipracil)
   b. Amoxicillin (Amoxil)
   c. Ceftriaxone (Rocephin)
   d. Cephradine (Anspor)

7. Trough serum drug levels for gentamicin should be drawn
   a. 5 minutes before the next dose.
   b. 15 minutes before the next dose.
   c. 2 hours before the next dose.
   d. 1 hour before the next dose.

8. Which of the following lab studies is indicative of nephrotoxicity?
   a. Elevated WBC
   b. Increased serum potassium
   c. Increased serum creatinine
   d. Elevated serum sodium

9. When administering aminoglycosides, concurrent administration of which of the following agents should be avoided because it may produce paralysis of respiratory muscles?
   a. Penicillin
   b. Propranolol (Inderal)
   c. Verapamil (Calan)
   d. Quinidine

10. Mr. J. has a peak gentamicin level of 14 µg/mL. This level is
    a. within the therapeutic range.
    b. lower than the therapeutic range.
    c. slightly above the therapeutic range.
    d. associated with nephrotoxicity.

■ Critical Thinking Case Study

Mrs. J. is being treated with tobramycin (Nebcin) for a *Pseudomonas* infection.

1. Identify the assessments that will be done before and during treatment with this drug.

Mrs. J.'s urinary output begins to drop.

2. Identify your nursing actions.

You speak to the physician on call about Mrs. J.'s decreased urinary output. He orders Lasix 80 mg IV push.

3. Discuss what you will do next.

CHAPTER 36

Tetracyclines, Sulfonamides, and Urinary Agents

■ Fill in the Blanks

Complete the following sentences.

1. Tetracyclines are effective against
_____ and _____
organisms as well as _____,
_____, some _____,
_____, and others.

2. The older tetracyclines are excreted mainly in
_____; the newer ones are excreted
mainly in _____.

3. Tetracyclines are the drugs of choice for

    a. _____.
    b. _____.
    c. _____.
    d. _____.
    e. _____.
    f. _____.
    g. _____.

4. _____ may be used in the management of _____ inappropriate ADH
secretion.

5. If tetracyclines are administered to children, they
can cause _____ and
_____.

6. Systemic sulfonamides are contraindicated during
_____, _____ and in
_____.

7. Sulfasalazine (Azulfidine) is contraindicated in
people who are _____ or who have
_____ or _____.

8. During sulfonamide therapy, fluids should be
forced to prevent _____.

9. With Mandelamine therapy, urine pH must be
_____. Urine can be acidified by
concomitant administration of
_____.

10. When taking tetracycline, you should avoid exposure to _____, _____,
and _____.

11. Oral tetracycline preparations should be administered _____.

12. Tetracyclines should not be administered with
_____.

13. Persons taking tetracycline should report the following symptoms to the physician:
_____, _____,
_____, _____,
_____, or itching in the
_____ area.

14. Sulfonamides _____, but do not
_____, bacteria.

15. Give nitrofurantoin (_____) for
_____ or _____ and
_____ UTIs.

16. Phenazopyridine (Pyridium) is a _____ that relieves
symptoms of _____,
_____, _____, and
_____.

17. Drugs that increase the effects of sulfonamides
include _____,
_____, and _____.

▪ Review Questions

1. You know your health teaching has been effective if your client, who is taking doxycycline (Vibramycin), states she should
   a. take the drug with food not containing metallic ions.
   b. contact the physician if she develops acne.
   c. only take it if she is going to be inside all day.
   d. take vitamin supplements with the medication.

2. If tetracycline is administered to children under 8 years of age, it can cause
   a. muscle weakness.
   b. renal insufficiency.
   c. gastrointestinal bleeding.
   d. permanent yellow-gray discoloration of the teeth.

3. Sulfisoxazole (Gantrisin) is prescribed for Mrs. P. What information should you give to Mrs. P.?
   a. "Since depression of bone can occur, take this drug for no more than 22 weeks."
   b. "Headache and dizziness are expected the first few days."
   c. "Be careful of over-the-counter medications because aspirin can increase toxicity of sulfonamides."
   d. "You must drink eight glasses of water daily when you take this drug."

4. Which of the following sulfonamides is used in the management of Crohn's disease?
   a. Sulfadiazine (Microsulfon)
   b. Sulfisoxazole (Gantrisin)
   c. Sulfamethoxazole-trimethoprim (Septra)
   d. Sulfasalazine (Azulfidine)

▪ Crossword Puzzle

ACROSS

4. The tetracycline most likely to cause photosensitivity.
5. May be used to treat *Pneumocystis carinii* pneumonia.
6. A topical sulfonamide used to treat burns.

DOWN

1. Available for ocular infections.
2. Used for ulcerative colitis.
3. Prevents bacterial colonization of wounds.

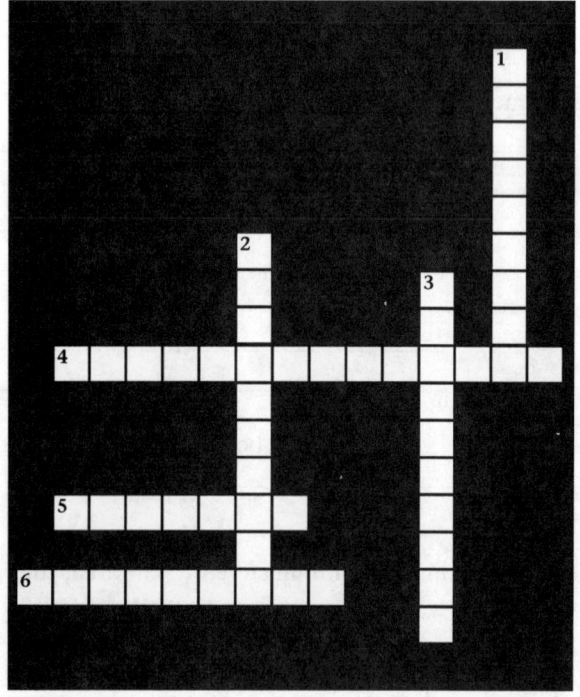

5. The only tetracycline that can be given safely to an individual who has renal impairment is
   a. minocycline (Minocin).
   b. oxytetracycline (Terramycin).
   c. methacycline (Rondomycin).
   d. doxycycline (Vibramycin).

6. Mrs. J., who is 6 months pregnant, comes to the doctor asking for a prescription for tetracycline to treat her acne. Your response should be
   a. "Tetracycline, if taken during pregnancy, will be deposited in the bones and teeth of the fetus."
   b. "Tetracycline can cause renal failure if taken during pregnancy."
   c. "The effect of tetracycline is decreased during pregnancy."
   d. "Taking tetracycline during pregnancy can cause premature labor."

7. When caring for a client taking tetracycline, you should assess him or her for symptoms of a super-infection, which include
   a. headache.
   b. sore mouth.
   c. decreased urinary output.
   d. blurred vision.

8. Which drug, if administered with a sulfonamide, will decrease its actions?
   a. Aspirin
   b. Propranolol (Inderal)
   c. Furosemide (Lasix)
   d. Maalox

9. When administering tetracycline, the nurse should observe Mr. C. for adverse effects of the medication, which include
   a. confusion.
   b. adrenal insufficiency.
   c. hepatotoxicity.
   d. elevated blood sugars.

10. Tetracycline is the drug of choice for treating
    a. typhus and cholera.
    b. respiratory tract infections.
    c. infections of the soft tissue.
    d. septicemia.

■ Critical Thinking Case Study

M.J., a 16-year-old high school student, comes to the dermatologist to be treated for acne. She is given a prescription for tetracycline.

1. Identify the assessments that will be done before she starts the medication.

2. Discuss the instructions you will give M.J. before she starts the medication.

M.J. returns to the office in 12 weeks and states that the medication has been ineffective.

3. Identify the information you will elicit from M.J. to help make your assessment.

After additional instructions, M.J. decides to continue the medication. She returns to the office 12 weeks later complaining of a sore throat.

4. Identify your nursing actions.

Macrolides and Miscellaneous Antibacterials

■ Fill in the Blanks

Complete the following sentences. At the end, identify the word or phrase formed by the boxed letter in each answer.

1. Newer macrolides cause less nausea, vomiting, and
   _ _ _ _ _ _ _ ☐.

2. Erthyomycin is used in clients who are allergic to
   _ _ _ _ _ _ _ _ _ ☐.

3. Azithromycin is prescribed for the treatment of urethritis caused by _ _ _ _ _ _ _ _ _ _
   ☐ _ _ _ _ _ _ _ _ _ _ _ organisms.

4. _ _ _ _ ☐ _ _ _ _ _ _ _ _ _ _ is used to treat *Helicobacter pylori* infections associated with peptic ulcer disease.

5. Erthyromycin is excreted in ☐ _ _ _ _ .

6. Chloramphenicol is effective against most gram-negative _ _ _ _ _ _ _ ☐.

7. *Mycobacterium avium* complex is an _ _ _ _ _
   _ _ _ _ _ _ _ _ ☐ infection that occurs mainly in people with HIV infection.

8. Chloramphenicol is the drug of choice for treating
   ☐ _ _ _ _ _ _ fever.

9. ☐ _ _ _ _ _ _ _ _ _ _ _ _ _, the prototype macrolide, is used infrequently because of microbial resistance.

10. Macrolides are widely used for ☐ _ _ _ _ _
    _ _ _ _ _ infections.

11. _ _ _ _ _ ☐ _ _ _ _ _ _ _ _ is used for treatment of gonococcal infections in people who are allergic to preferred drugs.

12. _ ☐ _ _ _ _ _ _ _ _ _ is used for treatment of *Clostridium difficile* infections associated with pseudomembranous colitis.

13. _ _ _ _ _ ☐ _ _ _ _, which include erthromycin, azithromycin, clarithromycin, and dirithromycin, have similar mechanisms of action.

■ Review Questions

1. The nurse should observe for this common adverse effect related to the administration of erythromycin.
   a. Vomiting
   b. Elevated blood sugar
   c. Elevated uric acid levels
   d. Decreased WBC

2. Which of the following medications will increase the effect of erythromycin when administered concurrently?
   a. Streptomycin
   b. Tetracycline
   c. Aztreonam (Azactam)
   d. Ceftriaxone (Rocephin)

3. Erythromycin is used as a substitute treatment for persons allergic to penicillin to treat
   a. glomerulonephritis.
   b. peritonitis.
   c. fungal infections.
   d. gonorrhea and syphilis.

4. A nursing measure that will help minimize the adverse effects associated with the administration of vancomycin is

   a. observe for convulsions, dizziness, and headaches.

   b. assess intake and output and serum creatinine levels.

   c. administer the medication over 4 hours.

   d. assess breath sounds during administration of the medication.

5. Phlebitis associated with the administration of IV erythromycin may be decreased by

   a. decreasing the amount of solution administered with the drug.

   b. applying warm compresses to the site during the infusion.

   c. diluting and administering the IV medication slowly.

   d. infusing the medication in 1000 cc of IV fluid over 8 hours.

6. The physician's order reads: "Administer clindamycin (Cleocin) 600 mg in 100 cc over 20 minutes." Using macrodrip tubing, (10 gtt = 1 cc), how fast will you run the IV?

   a. 20 gtt/minute

   b. 30 gtt/minute

   c. 40 gtt/minute

   d. 50 gtt/minute

7. Symptoms of pseudomembranous colitis that can result because of administration of clindamycin (Cleocin) include

   a. ascites and peripheral edema.

   b. hypertension and constipation.

   c. diarrhea, fever, and blood in stools.

   d. nausea, vomiting, and abdominal cramps.

8. M.J., who weighs 66 lb, is to receive clindamycin palmitate hydrochloride (Cleocin) in three divided doses. The maximum dose for a child her size is 15 mg/kg/day. If the pediatric Cleocin medication comes at 75 mg/mL, how many milliliters will M.J. receive per dose?

   a. 1 mL

   b. 2 mL

   c. 3 mL

   d. 4 mL

9. J.R., age 13, is being treated with clindamycin (Cleocin) for acne. Which of the following statements leads you to believe that he has understood the teaching you have done?

   a. "I can only take this drug for 2 weeks because it causes depression of bone growth."

   b. "Headache and dizziness are expected the first few days I take this medication."

   c. "I will report severe vomiting, diarrhea, or a rash to my physician."

   d. "I will drink eight glasses of water daily while I am taking this medication."

10. To decrease the potential for hypotension and flushing when administering vancomycin, you should

    a. administer an antihistamine prior to drug administration.

    b. dilute medication in 250 cc NS and administer over 2½ hours.

    c. place client in a supine position with legs elevated during administration.

    d. administer the medication slowly.

■ Critical Thinking Case Study

Mr. R., a 40-year-old attorney, has been experiencing chills, fever, and lethargy for 2 days. He is seen by his physician in the office, diagnosed with pneumonia, and started on erythromycin.

1. Identify the initial assessments the physician would have done to establish this diagnosis.

2. Identify the instructions that you will give Mr. R. before he returns home.

Mrs. R. calls you the next day to tell you that her husband has been vomiting on and off since he started on the medication.

3. Specify what your instruction to Mrs. R. will be.

Mr. R. is admitted to the hospital and started on erythromycin IV. He continues to vomit.

4. Identify what you will do.

CHAPTER 38

Drugs for Tuberculosis and *Mycobacterium Avium* Complex (MAC) Disease

■ Fill in the Blanks

Complete the following sentences.

1. Today, the recommended length of initial treatment for TB is _____ months.

2. The drugs used for initial treatment of TB are _____, _____, _____, and _____ or _____.

3. An indication for prophylactic use of INH would be a positive _____.

4. For persons exposed to someone with MDR-TB, _____ and _____ may be given.

5. The dosage of ethambutol is calculated according to _____.

6. Rifampin accelerates the _____ of other drugs by decreasing their _____ and _____.

7. Secondary tuberculosis drugs include
   _____ (_____),
   _____ (_____),
   _____ (_____), and
   _____ (_____).

8. The following reactions to antitubercular drugs should be reported to the physician:
   a. _____.
   b. _____.
   c. _____.
   d. _____.
   e. _____.
   f. _____.

■ Matching Exercise

Match each drug with the associated effects or information.

1. _____ INH (isoniazid)

2. _____ Rifampin

3. _____ Pyrazinamide

4. _____ Ethambutol

5. _____ Kanamycin

6. _____ Rifabutin

A. Causes a reddish-orange discoloration of body fluids.

B. Can affect red-green visual discrimination.

C. Accelerates the metabolism of several drugs.

D. Has antimycobacterial activity.

E. Can cause hepatotoxicity and peripheral neuropathy.

F. Causes hyperuricemia.

■ Identify the Treatment

Place an A in the table for drugs that are used alone to treat exposures to active TB and a C in the table for drugs that are used in combination. Use an asterisk to indicate that use of either drug is appropriate and a checkmark to indicate "may also be used."

	INH	Rifampin	Etham-butol	Pyrazin-amide	Ofloxacin	Strepto-mycin	Amikacin	Cipro-floxacin
1. Exposed to TB with a negative chest x-ray								
2. Exposed to TB that is INH resistant								
3. Exposed to MDR TB								
4. Initial diagnosis of active TB								
5. Active MDR TB								
6. Active TB during pregnancy								

■ Review Questions

1. What findings would lead you to believe that your client may be experiencing hepatic toxicity from isoniazid (INH)?
   a. Diarrhea
   b. Numbness and tingling
   c. Visual disturbances
   d. Dark urine

2. Which of the following drugs should be taken on an empty stomach to prevent delayed absorption?
   a. Rifampin (Rifadin)
   b. Para-amino salicylic acid (PAS)
   c. Isoniazid (INH)
   d. Streptomycin

3. When taking INH, hepatitis and liver damage may occur
   a. 72 hours after initiation of drug therapy.
   b. during the first 8 weeks of drug therapy.
   c. a week to 10 days after initiation of drug therapy.
   d. between the sixth and ninth months of drug therapy.

4. Which of the following statements by your client, who has active TB, leads you to believe that she has a good understanding of how she is to take the medication?
   a. "I will take the medication until the symptoms subside."
   b. "I may have to take as many as four medications for 4 months."
   c. "I will take the medication for 6 months and then I am finished."
   d. "I will take a combination of medications for 9 months to 2 years."

5. Which of the following statements is true regarding tuberculosis?
   a. Symptoms of TB occur within 2 weeks of exposure.
   b. TB affects only the lungs.
   c. TB can be controlled by chemotherapy.
   d. TB can be cured with radiation therapy.

6. Clients receiving INH should be assessed monthly for symptoms of hepatitis, which include
   a. brown urine and bruising.
   b. weight gain and abdominal distension.
   c. peripheral edema and tachycardia.
   d. nausea, fatigue, and jaundice.

7. When taking isoniazid (INH), which of the following things should Mr. C. be instructed to avoid?

    a. Alcohol

    b. Caffeine

    c. Dairy products

    d. Citrus fruits

8. You are doing the discharge teaching of a person newly diagnosed with TB. You need to tell him that the usual length of time that persons must take isoniazid (INH) is

    a. 10 days.

    b. 3 months.

    c. 6 months.

    d. 1 year.

9. Mr. J. weighs 143 lb and the recommended daily dose of ethambutol (Myambutol) is 15 mg/kg/day. How many milligrams should he receive daily?

    a. 500 mg

    b. 650 mg

    c. 975 mg

    d. 1250 mg

10. Which of the following statements by Mrs. G. leads you to believe that she has understood the teaching you have done regarding rifampin (Rifadin)?

    a. "Dizziness, drowsiness, and decreased urinary output are common with this drug, but they will subside over time."

    b. "Constipation will be a problem, so I will increase the fiber in my diet."

    c. "Initially, I may experience blurred vision and inability to distinguish colors, but it will improve in a few weeks."

    d. "This medication may cause my bodily secretions to turn red."

■ Critical Thinking Case Study

Ms. G., a 25-year-old public health nurse, has a positive tuberculin test but a negative chest x-ray. She is started on INH.

1. Identify what your instruction will be for Ms. G.

Ms. G. calls the office 5 months after starting the medication, and states that she has stopped menstruating and that her skin has a yellow cast.

2. Identify your response.

Study Guide to Accompany Clinical Drug Therapy: Rationales for Nursing Practice, sixth edition, by Gail Ropelewski-Ryan.

CHAPTER 39

Antiviral Drugs

■ True or False

1. _____ Viruses can live for hours outside of a living organism.

2. _____ Acyclovir (Zovirax) inactivates the herpesvirus and prevents the recurrence of the disease.

3. _____ Amantadine (Symmetrel) may be useful in the treatment of influenza A infections.

4. _____ Ganciclovir (Cytovene) is effective in preventing CMV retinitis in persons with organ transplants.

5. _____ Ribavirin (Virazole) is administered by inhalation for the treatment of RSV infection.

6. _____ Zidovudine (AZT) was the first anti-HIV drug developed.

7. _____ Stavudine may be used with didanosine to prevent peripheral neuropathy.

8. _____ Ophthalmic antiviral preparations such as trifluridine can cause ocular toxicity.

9. _____ Persons who have visible herpes lesions will not spread the disease if they apply acyclovir before having sexual intercourse.

10. _____ There are many vaccines available that will prevent viral diseases, including poliomyelitis, mumps, yellow fever, and rabies.

11. _____ Zidovudine (AZT), when used for persons with AIDS, prevents the occurrence of opportunistic infections.

12. _____ Viral infections can occur without any signs and symptoms of illness.

13. _____ Repeated courses of acyclovir (Zovirax) therapy may result in severe anemia and granulocytopenia.

14. _____ Seizures are associated with high plasma levels of amantadine (Symmetrel).

15. _____ Nevirapine induces drug-metabolizing enzymes in the liver.

■ Matching Exercise

TERMS AND CONCEPTS

Match each drug with the adverse effects associated with it.

1. _____ Indinavir (Crixivan)

2. _____ Amprenavir (Agenerase)

3. _____ Nevirapine (Viramune)

4. _____ Nelfinavir (Viracept)

5. _____ Delavirdine (Rescriptor)

6. _____ Zalcitabine (Hivid)

A. Serous skin reactions

B. Diarrhea

C. Nausea and skin rash

D. Hepatotoxicity

E. Kidney stones

F. Peripheral neuropathy

■ Review Questions

1. Adverse effects of acyclovir (Zovirax) that the nurse needs to assess for include

   a. increased serum creatinine.

   b. thrombocytopenia.

   c. respiratory distress.

   d. psychosis.

2. An expected outcome after the administration of acyclovir (Zovirax) for genital herpes is

   a. decreased fever.

   b. decreased pain.

   c. prevention of recurrence.

   d. smaller size of lesion during next exacerbation.

3. Live attenuated viral vaccines should not be administered to persons who are receiving

   a. oral hypoglycemic agents.

   b. antineoplastic agents.

   c. intravenous antibiotics.

   d. pulmonary bronchodilators.

4. Which of the following statements by Mr. J. leads you to believe that he understands how to use trifluridine (Viroptic)?

   a. "After I take this medication, I may notice burning, stinging, or eyelid edema."

   b. "Each time after I administer the medication, I will apply cold compresses to my eyes."

   c. "I should use this drug for no longer than 10 days because it can cause ocular toxicity."

   d. "I will use the medication once a day before I go to bed."

5. Which of the following statements by your client with AIDS leads you to believe that he needs additional teaching?

   a. "Zidovudine (AZT) may need to be stopped temporarily if bone marrow depression occurs."

   b. "Zidovudine (AZT) therapy may result in the development of anemia."

   c. "Zidovudine (AZT) slows the progression of the disease but does not cure it."

   d. "Zidovudine (AZT) prevents the transmission of the virus through sexual contact."

6. Ribavirin (Virazole) for treatment of respiratory syncytial viral infections is administered via

   a. the rectum.

   b. an intravenous route.

   c. subcutaneous injection.

   d. inhalation.

7. You are to administer acyclovir (Zovirax) intravenously. The recommended dose is 5 mg/kg q8h. Your client weighs 110 lb. How much medication will you administer per day?

   a. 250 mg

   b. 500 mg

   c. 750 mg

   d. 1000 mg

8. For which of the following disorders in Mr. G.'s history would you contact the doctor before administering amantadine (Symmetrel)?

   a. Allergies to pollen and dog dander

   b. Epilepsy

   c. Diabetes mellitus

   d. Chronic lung disease

9. Which of the following medications, if administered concurrently with zidovudine (AZT), will increase its effects?

   a. Acetaminophen (Tylenol)

   b. Atropine

   c. Amphotericin B

   d. Propranolol (Inderal)

10. Which of the following medications, if administered with amantadine (Symmetrel), will cause blurred vision, dry mouth, and urine retention?

    a. Atropine

    b. Furosemide (Lasix)

    c. Prednisone

    d. Sodium bicarbonate

■ Critical Thinking Case Study

J.J., a 32-year-old man, has recently been diagnosed with HIV infection and is started on zidovudine (AZT).

1. Discuss the instructions that you will give him.

2. Identify three nursing diagnoses that would be appropriate for J.J.

J.J.'s disease progresses rapidly. Within 3 years, he develops AIDS and has contracted several opportunistic infections. He is presently being seen for cytomegalovirus retinitis, for which the doctor orders ganciclovir (Cytovene).

3. Discuss the instructions that you will give him.

J.J. calls you because he has noticed some bleeding. He is crying on the phone and states, "I don't want to die."

4. Discuss how you will respond to J.J.

CHAPTER 40

Antifungal Drugs

■ Matching Exercise

TERMS AND CONCEPTS

Match the concept with the term for it.

1. _____ Tinea pedis.

2. _____ Ringworm of the scalp.

3. _____ Thrush.

4. _____ This can occur as a nosocomial infection in patients with serious illnesses.

5. _____ Found in soil and organic debris.

6. _____ Causes a respiratory infection that resembles pneumonia or tuberculosis.

7. _____ Used to treat fungal infections of the eye.

8. _____ Drug used to treat athlete's foot.

9. _____ Can cause hypokalemia and anemia.

10. _____ Drug administered topically to treat dermatophytosis.

11. _____ Adverse effects of this drug include nausea, vomiting, jaundice, and abdominal pain.

12. _____ This drug may cause photosensitivity.

13. _____ The length of time Amphotericin B is administered.

14. _____ Signs and symptoms of histoplasmosis, coccidioidomycosis, and blastomycosis.

15. _____ A drug used for the treatment of vaginal candidiasis.

16. _____ Fungi that cause superficial skin infections.

17. _____ Can occur following inhalation of airborne spores from air conditioning units.

18. _____ This drug will increase the effects of fluconazole.

19. _____ Notify health care provider if client receiving fluconazole (Diflucan) has these symptoms.

20. _____ Clients who work in gardens or plant nurseries are at risk.

A. Athlete's foot
B. Amphotericin B (Fungizone)
C. Blastomycosis
D. Miconazole (Monistat)
E. Haloprogin (Halotex)
F. Oral candidiasis
G. Tinea capitis
H. Natamycin (Natacyn)
I. Fungus causing histoplasmosis
J. Systemic candidiasis
K. Griseofulvin (Fulvicin)
L. Sporotrichosis
M. 6–12 weeks
N. Cough, fever, malaise
O. Ketoconazole (Nizoral)
P. Abdominal pain, fever, jaundice
Q. Clotrimazole (Lotrimin)
R. Aspergillosis
S. Dermatophytes
T. Hydrochlorothiazide

Study Guide to Accompany Clinical Drug Therapy: Rationales for Nursing Practice, sixth edition, by Gail Ropelewski-Ryan.

■ Fill in the Blanks

Complete the following sentences.

1. Mechanisms of contracting a fungal infection include _____, _____, and _____.

2. Drugs used for superficial fungal infections of the skin are usually administered _____.

3. Exposure to pigeon, chicken, or bat excreta can result in _____.

4. Corticosteroid use can lead to a _____ infection.

5. _____ is a potent intravenous antifungal drug used for serious systemic infections.

■ Review Questions

1. The drug used to treat tinea pedis is
   a. acrisorcin (Akrinol).
   b. haloprogin (Halotex).
   c. griseofulvin (Fulvicin).
   d. nystatin (Mycostatin).

2. Your client weighs 88 lb and is to receive amphotericin B (Fungizone) 0.50 mg/kg daily. If she receives two doses daily, how much medication will she receive per dose?
   a. 10 mg
   b. 20 mg
   c. 100 mg
   d. 200 mg

3. Which of the following medications, if administered concurrently with amphotericin B, may increase nephrotoxicity?
   a. Aminoglycosides
   b. Antipyretics
   c. Beta-adrenergic blockers
   d. Potassium-sparing diuretics

4. Your client is receiving intravenous amphotericin B (Fungizone). He should be observed for
   a. tachycardia.
   b. an elevated serum creatinine level.
   c. a low serum sodium level.
   d. severe diarrhea.

5. Which of the following statements leads you to believe that your client has understood the teaching you have done regarding ketoconazole (Nizoral)?
   a. "I should take this medication with milk or an antacid to prevent gastrointestinal upset."
   b. "I know that as a result of taking this medication, I could develop nausea, vomiting, and abdominal pain."
   c. "I know that I will need to take this medication for a week to 10 days, but no longer."
   d. "I know that as a result of taking this medication, I could develop a resistance to this medication."

6. Which of the following medications, if administered concurrently with griseofulvin (Fulvicin), will decrease its effect?
   a. Cephalothin (Keflin)
   b. Furosemide (Lasix)
   c. Prednisone
   d. Phenobarbital

7. Which of the following is a drug used to treat histoplasmosis?
   a. Acrisorcin (Akrinol)
   b. Flucytosine (Ancobon)
   c. Natamycin (Natacyn)
   d. Ketoconazole (Nizoral)

8. Which of the following instructions will you give your client regarding administration of ciclopirox (Loprox)?
   a. "Apply the ointment to the lesions for 3 months."
   b. "Apply the medication to the skin lesions twice a day for 2–4 weeks."
   c. "Place the solution in a sitz bath and soak in it twice daily."
   d. "Fill the applicator with the medication, apply the cream q4h, and place sterile pads on the lesions after each treatment."

9. Which of the following statements by M.S. leads you to believe that she has understood the teaching you have done regarding the use of natamycin (Natacyn) for a fungal infection of her eye?

   a. "I will apply one drop to each eye q 1–2 hours for 3 days, then every 3–4 hours for 2–3 weeks."

   b. "I will take the medication orally, on an empty stomach, twice a day for 2 to 4 weeks."

   c. "After each application of the medication, I will apply cool compresses to my eyes."

   d. "I will rinse my eyes with the solution four times a day for 1 month."

10. Which of the following instructions should you give your client who is being treated with econazole (Spectazole) for ringworm?

    a. "Wash your head four times every day for 2 weeks."

    b. "Do not share towels with any other member of the family."

    c. "Do not eat meat while using this medication."

    d. "Comb the medication into your hair, then apply gauze over your head to keep from spreading it to the others."

■ Critical Thinking Case Study

M., a 32-year-old model, comes to the physician's office with a fungal infection of her fingernails caused by application of ceramic fingernails. The physician orders griseofulvin (Fulvicin). M. is leaving for a job in Hawaii and asks for a 4-week supply of the medication.

1. Discuss with M. why her plans concern you.

2. Identify the instructions that you will give M., including the adverse effects of griseofulvin (Fulvicin).

3. Identify three nursing diagnoses for M.

M. returns after her trip to Hawaii complaining of headache, dizziness, and fatigue.

4. Identify what you will do.

CHAPTER 41

Antiparasitics

■ True or False

1. _____ *Entamoeba histolytica* can live outside of the body for long periods.

2. _____ Amebiasis can result in abscesses of the lungs and brain.

3. _____ Malaria is a common cause of mortality and morbidity worldwide.

4. _____ Giardiasis is transmitted by the ingestion of improperly cooked beef, pork, or fish.

5. _____ Roundworms, caused by *Ascaris lumbricoides*, are the most common parasitic worm infections in the United States.

6. _____ Scabies and pediculosis can be transmitted by direct contact with the personal effects of an infected person.

7. _____ Parasitic worms can enter the bloodstream and migrate to other body tissues.

8. _____ Metronidazole stains feces a bright red color that can be mistaken for blood.

9. _____ Lindane (Kwell), used for the treatment of scabies, is absorbed through the skin and can produce CNS toxicity.

10. _____ Pyrimethamine (Daraprim) is used to treat malaria attacks.

11. _____ Visible skin lesions associated with scabies are commonly found between the fingers.

12. _____ Topical antitrichomonal agents can cause rash and inflammation.

13. _____ When a *Trichomonas* infection is diagnosed, it is common practice to treat the sexual partner as well as the individual with the confirmed diagnosis.

14. _____ Quinine can also be used for treatment of nocturnal leg cramps.

15. _____ A person being treated for dwarf tapeworms with niclosamide (Niclocide) is not considered cured until he or she has had negative stools for 3 months.

16. _____ Toxoplasmosis may be caused by contact with feces from infected cats.

■ Review Questions

1. Mr. C. is being treated for amebiasis. The nurse should instruct him that the following adverse reactions are commonly experienced with amebicides:

   a. tachycardia and hypotension.

   b. oliguria and weight gain.

   c. nausea, vomiting, and diarrhea.

   d. dizziness and paresthesias.

2. The drug of choice for prevention and treatment of *Pneumocystis carinii* pneumonia (PCP) is

   a. trimethoprim-sulfamethoxazole (Bactrim).

   b. trimetrexate (Neutrexin).

   c. mebendazole (Vermox).

   d. pyrantel (Antiminth).

3. Which of the following instructions should you give to Ms. G., who is starting on a douche for trichomoniasis?

   a. "Administer the douche daily for 1 month."

   b. "Administer the douche three times a day for 1 week."

   c. "Avoid sexual intercourse during treatment so that you can be sure you are free of infection."

   d. "Wear gloves when administering the douche and keep it away from your perineal area."

4. P.G. is sent home with a note from school stating that she has pediculosis (head lice). Which of the following instructions should you give P.G.'s mother about the use of permethrin (Nix)?

    a. "Apply to P.G.'s head three times a day for 2 weeks."

    b. "Bathe P.G., apply Nix to all her body surfaces, leave it on for 24 hours, and bathe her again."

    c. "Apply it to her scalp and hair; leave it on for 10 minutes, then rinse off with water."

    d. "Have P.G. take a warm shower in the morning and apply Nix all over her body; rinse off that evening."

5. Which of the following statements by a client being treated for pinworms leads you to believe that she has understood the teaching you have done regarding mebendazole (Vermox)?

    a. "I will need to have three negative stool cultures before I will be considered free of the pinworms."

    b. "I may continue to expel worms for 3 days after therapy is completed."

    c. "I will not drink alcohol when I am using this medication."

    d. "I will eat foods high in roughage to assist with passage of the worms."

6. Which of the following drugs, if taken with chloroquine phosphate (Aralen), will decrease its effects?

    a. Vitamin C (ascorbic acid)

    b. Vitamin E (Aquasol E)

    c. Furosemide (Lasix)

    d. Cephradine (Velosef)

7. When quinine is administered, you should observe for signs of cinchonism, which include

    a. skin rash and unpleasant taste.

    b. hypocalcemia and vertigo.

    c. headache, tinnitus, and blurred vision.

    d. nausea, vomiting, and diarrhea.

8. Your client is diagnosed with trichomoniasis and started on metronidazole (Flagyl). Which of the following instructions should you give her?

    a. "Change your bed linens daily until the infection is gone."

    b. "Your partner should also be treated to prevent the possibility of reinfection."

    c. "You should refrain from sexual intercourse for 2 months."

    d. "You may gain 2–5 lb while on this medication, but you will lose the weight as soon as the medication is discontinued."

9. Mr. B. is receiving aerosol pentamidine (NebuPent) for prophylaxis for *Pneumocystis carinii* pneumonia (PCP). He should be observed for adverse reactions to this medication, which include

    a. hypertension, tachycardia, and diarrhea.

    b. headache, tinnitus, and blurred vision.

    c. chest pain, dyspnea, and dizziness.

    d. weakness, constipation, and paresthesia.

10. Your client is taking metronidazole (Flagyl) for trichomoniasis. Which of the following statements leads you to believe that she has understood the teaching you have done?

    a. "I will limit my intake of caffeine while I am taking this medication."

    b. "I will eat a diet low in sodium while taking this medication."

    c. "I will increase my daily intake of potassium while taking this medication."

    d. "I will not drink any alcohol while taking this medication."

CHAPTER 42

Physiology of the Hematopoietic and Immune Systems

■ Matching Exercise

TERMS AND CONCEPTS

Match the concept with the term for it.

1. _____ A generalized reaction to cellular injury from any cause.

2. _____ Stimulates production of antibodies that destroy foreign invaders.

3. _____ Detects and eliminates foreign substances that may cause tissue injury.

4. _____ Develops during gestation or after birth; may be active or passive.

5. _____ Occurs when antibodies are formed by the immune system of another person or animal and transferred to the host.

6. _____ Foreign substances that initiate immune responses.

7. _____ WBCs found throughout the body in lymphoid tissues.

8. _____ The first WBCs that start phagocytosis.

9. _____ WBCs that arrive later, ingest larger amounts of antigen, and have a longer life span than the first WBCs that respond.

10. _____ The primary regulator of the immune response.

11. _____ Originate in stem cells in bone marrow.

12. _____ Protein growth factors secreted by WBCs that stimulate leukocyte replication and function.

13. _____ Interfere with the ability of viruses to replicate in infected cells.

14. _____ Stimulate growth and differentiation of cells.

15. _____ A factor that affects immunologic response.

A. Immune response
B. Passive immunity
C. Antigens
D. Inflammation
E. Immune cells
F. T lymphocytes
G. Interferons
H. Immune system
I. Cytokines
J. Acquired immunity
K. Interleukins
L. Monocytes
M. Age
N. B lymphocytes
O. Neutrophils

■ Review Questions

1. Active immunity
   a. occurs when antibodies are formed by the immune system of another person and transferred to the host.
   b. develops within 6 months after birth.
   c. occurs when foreign substances stimulate the production of antibodies.
   d. develops as a result of antibodies that are innate to the organism being stimulated to produce WBCs.

2. When there is cellular injury, which of the following WBCs arrives first and begins phagocytosis?
   a. Lymphocytes
   b. Basophils
   c. Monocytes
   d. Neutrophils

3. Interleukins
   a. stimulate B lymphocyte activity.
   b. interfere with multiplication of stem cells.
   c. stimulate growth and differentiation of lymphoid cells into lymphocytes.
   d. interfere with the ability of viruses in infected cells to replicate.

4. The function of colony-stimulating factors (CSF) is to
   a. stimulate growth of blood cells.
   b. suppress T-cell production.
   c. inhibit protein production.
   d. stimulate production of antibodies.

5. Natural killer cells act by
   a. releasing powerful chemicals that kill infectious microorganisms.
   b. binding to antigens and damaging their cell membrane.
   c. injecting fluid into the antigen cell, causing edema and death.
   d. decreasing the activities of the B cells.

6. Which of the following immunoglobulins crosses the placenta to provide maternal acquired antibodies to the infant?
   a. IgG
   b. IgA
   c. IgM
   d. IgE

7. T lymphocyte growth factor (TGF)
   a. promotes wound healing and bone remodeling.
   b. interferes with the multiplication of stem cells.
   c. stimulates the production of erythrocytes.
   d. interferes with the ability of viruses to replicate.

8. A lack of which of the following decreases the number and function of T cells?
   a. Calcium
   b. Protein
   c. Potassium
   d. Fluid volume

9. Substances that interact with immune cells to induce the immune response are
   a. antigens.
   b. antibodies.
   c. cytokines.
   d. monocytes.

10. Which of the following depresses immune function and increases the risk of developing an infection?
   a. Heart disease
   b. Use of beta-adrenergic blockers
   c. Dehydration
   d. Stress

CHAPTER 43

Immunizing Agents

■ Fill in the Blanks

Complete the following sentences.

1. Active immunity develops as a result of exposure to an _____ to induce _____.

2. Passive immunity occurs when _____ are transferred to the host.

3. Vaccines are suspensions of microorganisms that have been _____, or _____.

4. Toxoids are bacterial toxins that have been modified to destroy _____.

5. The following vaccines are not routinely administered to Americans unless they are traveling abroad:

   a. _____.
   b. _____.
   c. _____.
   d. _____.
   e. _____.
   f. _____.
   g. _____.
   h. _____.

6. Vaccines and toxoids are contraindicated during
   _____, _____,
   _____, and _____.

7. If your client experiences an allergic reaction from the administration of an immunizing agent, _____ should be administered immediately.

8. Persons receiving a DTP injection may experience _____ and _____ at the injection site. They should be instructed to take _____ for symptomatic relief.

9. _____ (_____) is a rare reaction to oral poliovirus vaccine.

10. Annual _____ and one-time _____ vaccine are recommended for healthy older adults.

■ Exercise on Immunization

ADMINISTRATION OF IMMUNIZATIONS

Specify how each immunization is administered.

1. _____ Measles vaccine.

2. _____ Hepatitis B vaccine.

3. _____ Poliovirus vaccine.

4. _____ Tetanus toxoid.

Schedule for Immunization of Infants and Children

Place an x in the table to identify the appropriate timing(s) for immunizations, based upon recommendations from the Advisory Committee on Immunization Practices (ACIP), the American Academy of Pediatrics (AAP), and the American Academy of Family Physicians (AAFP).

	Birth	1 mo	2 mo	4 mo	6 mo	10-12 mo	15 mo	18 mo	4-6 yr	11-12 yr	Every 10 yr	14-16
Polio (IPV)												
Diphtheria-tetanus-pertussis (DTP)												
Diphtheria-tetanus (DT)												
Measles-mumps-rubella (MMR)												
Haemophilus influenza Type B (Hib)												
Hepatitis B (HBV)												
Varicella zoster (Var) chicken pox												

■ Review Questions

1. When administering DTP to an 18-month-old child, you should give the parents the following instructions:
   a. "Apply cold compresses to the injection site."
   b. "Do not let A.J. walk on her leg for 2 hours."
   c. "Take A.J. home and give her a warm bath and massage her leg."
   d. "Give Tylenol q4–6h because fever is a common adverse reaction to this medication."

2. Persons who have been immunized can develop serum sickness. The symptoms are
   a. laryngeal edema and urticaria.
   b. severe respiratory distress and tachycardia.
   c. fever, arthralgia, and enlarged lymph nodes.
   d. somnolence, convulsions, and dizziness.

3. Mrs. J. tells you that the last time her child received a DTP immunization he had a fever of 104.5°F. Identify your nursing action.
   a. Withhold the immunization and contact the physician.
   b. Administer diphenhydramine hydrochloride (Benadryl) before administration of DTP.
   c. Administer only a DT immunization.
   d. Administer acetaminophen (Tylenol) with the DTP.

4. Mrs. J.'s child has been bitten by a rabid raccoon. Which of these statements leads you to believe that she understands how the rabies vaccine is to be administered?
   a. "My child will receive five IM doses of this drug: one today, then 3 days, 7 days, 14 days, and 28 days later."
   b. "My child must receive a daily injection for 4 weeks."
   c. "My child will receive an initial injection followed by an oral drug for 2 months."
   d. "My child will receive a SC injection every 4 weeks for four doses, then a booster 6 months after the last dose."

5. MMR (measles, mumps, and rubella) vaccination is contraindicated in
   a. persons with lung disease.
   b. persons who have had chicken pox.
   c. children under the age of five.
   d. women who are pregnant.

6. Drugs that alter the effects of vaccines include
   a. antacids.
   b. corticosteroids.
   c. thiazide diuretics.
   d. beta-adrenergic blockers.

7. Anaphylaxis resulting from the administration of an immunizing agent can be effectively treated with
   a. promethazine hydrochloride (Phenergan).
   b. diphenhydramine hydrochloride (Benadryl).
   c. epinephrine (Adrenalin).
   d. prednisone (Deltasone).

8. Vaccines provide
   a. active immunity.
   b. passive immunity.
   c. natural immunity.
   d. cell-mediated immunity.

9. Vaccines should not be given to children if they
   a. have a febrile illness.
   b. are diabetic.
   c. have a seizure disorder.
   d. weigh less than 20 lb.

10. If an individual is going to experience an allergic reaction to an immunization, it will usually occur within
    a. 3–5 minutes after administration.
    b. 30 minutes after administration.
    c. 3–5 hours after administration.
    d. 2–3 days after administration.

■ Critical Thinking Case Study

S., a 6-month-old infant, has come to the clinic to receive her immunizations. Her mother states that S. had a reaction after her last immunization and that she does not want S. to have any more immunizations.

1. Identify what questions you should ask the mother.

S.'s mother finally agrees to allow the infant to have the immunization.

3. Identify what assessment should be done before administering the DTP and for what reasons you would withhold an immunization.

S.'s mother calls the office to report that S. has a lump on her leg where she received the immunization.

4. Describe the advice you would give S.'s mother.

2. Identify the information you should give S.'s mother regarding immunizations.

CHAPTER 44

Hematopoietic and Immunostimulant Drugs

■ Matching Exercise

TERMS AND CONCEPTS

Match the concept with the term for it.

1. _____ A drug that stimulates production of RBCs.

2. _____ Used to treat bone marrow graft failure.

3. _____ Decreased production of neutrophils.

4. _____ Used with persons undergoing bone marrow transplantation.

5. _____ Approved for the treatment of Kaposi's sarcoma.

6. _____ Approved for the treatment of renal cell carcinoma.

7. _____ An immunizing agent against tuberculosis, also used for bladder cancer.

8. _____ Normal white blood count.

9. _____ A mood-stabilizing agent that mobilizes neutrophils and is sometimes given to persons with chemotherapy-induced neutropenia.

10. _____ Stimulates platelet production.

A. 5000–10,000/mm^3

B. Epoetin alfa (Epogen)

C. 15,000–25,000/mm^3

D. Filgrastim (Neupogen)

E. Bacillus Calmette-Guérin (BCG)

F. Neutropenia

G. Interleukin-2 (aldesleukin)

H. Oprelvekin (Neumega)

I. Interferon alfa-2b

J. Sargramostim

K. Lithium

■ True or False

1. _____ Interferons can only be administered by injection.

2. _____ Immunostimulants are used exclusively for persons with cancer.

3. _____ Interferons should not be administered to persons who have hepatitis.

4. _____ Toxicity from the administration of interleukin-2 (aldesleukin) can result in hard-to-control seizures.

5. _____ Isolation procedures must be instituted if the neutrophil count drops below 500/mm^3.

■ Crossword Puzzle

ACROSS

1. Any previous infections should be resolved before beginning therapy with this drug.

3. This type of drug is given only by injection.

4. Low _____ count places the patient at risk of infection.

6. Interferon alfa-2b is approved for treatment of recurring _____.

8. Stimulates granulocyte production.

9. An abnormal decrease in white blood cells.

DOWN

2. Given after bone marrow transplantation via slow IV.

5. Abbreviation for the immunostimulant that can cause bladder cancer remission.

7. This type of tumor in the breast, lung, or colon does not respond to interferon.

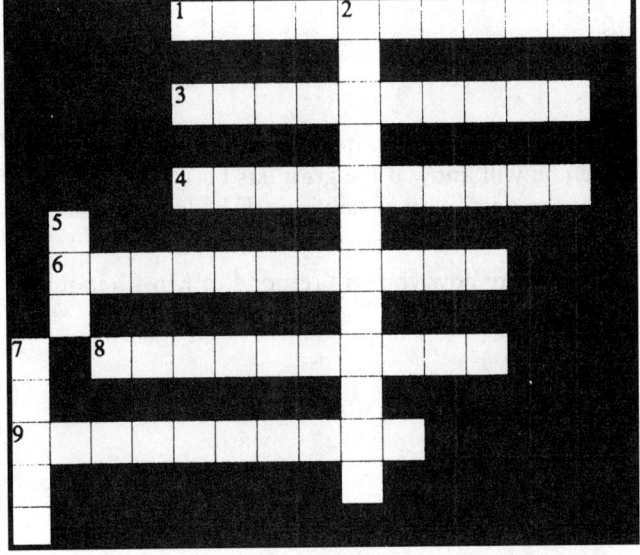

■ Review Questions

1. Your client is receiving filgrastim and complains of bone pain. You should

   a. administer a nonsteroidal anti-inflammatory drug.

   b. stop the drug immediately.

   c. apply warm compresses to his arms and legs.

   d. assist him with passive range-of-motion exercises of his extremities.

2. Which of the following drugs, if administered concurrently with interleukin-2 (aldesleukin), will decrease its effects?

   a. Prednisone

   b. Propranolol (Inderal)

   c. Ibuprofen (Motrin)

   d. Gentamicin (Garamycin)

3. The following lab studies should be done daily during interleukin-2 (aldesleukin) therapy?

   a. ABGs and O₂ saturations

   b. PT and APTT

   c. Blood glucose

   d. Electrolytes, liver and renal function tests

4. The following lab work should be done routinely during immunostimulant therapy:

   a. PT and PTT.

   b. hematocrit and hemoglobin.

   c. CBC, WBC, and platelet count.

   d. creatinine clearance.

5. After bone marrow transplant, the engrafted cells will mature and begin to produce blood cells in

   a. 2–4 hours.

   b. 2–4 days.

   c. 2–4 weeks.

   d. 2–4 months.

6. Sargramostin (Leukine) helps to

   a. normalize platelet counts.

   b. increase hemoglobin levels.

   c. decrease the risk of infection.

   d. enhance red blood cell production.

7. Bacillus Calmette-Guérin (BCG), used to treat bladder cancers, is
   a. administered by inhalation.
   b. applied via applicator in gel form.
   c. administered parenterally over 12 hours.
   d. instilled into the bladder.

8. The expected outcome of administering epoetin alfa (Epogen) to a client with chronic renal failure is
   a. decreased bleeding.
   b. increased WBC production.
   c. decreased secretion of renin.
   d. increased RBC production.

9. The administration of interferons may be stopped if the client experiences
   a. ankle edema.
   b. nausea and vomiting.
   c. diarrhea.
   d. difficulty breathing.

10. Which of the following medications should be administered with epoetin alfa (Epogen)?
    a. Aspirin
    b. Antacids
    c. Iron
    d. Prednisone

■ Critical Thinking Case Study

Mr. J., a 36-year-old accountant, is to receive a bone marrow transplant. He will be receiving sargramostim after the procedure to help prevent graft failure.

1. Discuss the teaching that you will do with Mr. J. and his wife.

2. Identify the assessments that you will do.

Mr. J. is very nervous after the transplant and asks you when he will know if the graft has been successful and what the possibility of failure is. (The learner will need additional sources to answer the question below.)

3. Identify how you will respond to Mr. J.'s inquiry.

CHAPTER 45

Immunosuppressants

■ True or False

1. _____ Rheumatoid arthritis results from an inappropriate activation of the immune response.

2. _____ Acute organ rejection occurs within 2 days following transplantation.

3. _____ Once an individual has had a transplanted organ for a year, he or she will not experience organ rejection.

4. _____ Corticosteroids increase the numbers of circulating basophils, eosinophils, and monocytes.

5. _____ Cytotoxic antimetabolites block cellular reproduction.

6. _____ Methotrexate (Rheumatrex) has been used to treat severe psoriasis.

7. _____ Cyclosporine (Sandimmune) is used to prevent graft versus host disease in bone marrow transplant recipients.

8. _____ Antithymocyte globulin (ATG) should not be administered to persons who have an allergy to cow serum.

9. _____ Isolation techniques are instituted for transplant recipients whose neutrophil count drops below $1000/mm^3$.

10. _____ If immunosuppression is excessive, graft versus host disease can occur.

11. _____ Immunosuppressive drugs increase the production of T cells.

12. _____ Lymphoma may result from immunosuppression.

13. _____ A disadvantage of tacrolimus versus cyclosporine is that more corticosteroid therapy and a long hospital stay are needed.

14. _____ The preferred route for administering cyclosporine (Sandimmune) is intramuscular because it is more effective.

15. _____ Symptoms of neurotoxicity produced by cyclosporine include confusion, hallucinations, and seizures.

■ Review Questions

1. Mr. P. is receiving methotrexate after a transplant. Methotrexate is also effective for which one of the following inflammatory disorders?
   a. Psoriasis
   b. Lupus erythematosus
   c. Acne
   d. Herpes zoster

2. Persons receiving azathioprine after a kidney transplant should be observed for
   a. neurotoxicity.
   b. bone marrow depression.
   c. liver toxicity.
   d. renal failure.

3. Your client asks you how methotrexate (Rheumatrex) works in autoimmune disorders. The best reply would be, "It...
   a. decreases production and function of T cells."
   b. inhibits the production of neutrophils."
   c. reduces the concentration of WBCs."
   d. prevents the formation of antigens."

4. A person receiving immunosuppressants after bone marrow transplantation should be assessed for graft versus host disease (GVHD). Symptoms include

    a. elevated alkaline phosphatase, transaminase, and bilirubin levels.

    b. a 5–10 point drop in hematocrit and hemoglobin.

    c. peripheral edema and decreased urinary output.

    d. elevated serum potassium, sodium, and calcium levels.

5. Children receiving corticosteroids to suppress immune reactions need to be told that this can result in

    a. pigmentation changes.

    b. hair loss.

    c. growth retardation.

    d. renal failure.

6. Cushingoid symptoms that can result from long-term administration of corticosteroids include the development of

    a. alopecia.

    b. a buffalo hump.

    c. peripheral edema.

    d. dysrhythmia.

7. Immunosuppressive drugs are used to inactivate T cells, which

    a. stimulate B cells to produce antibodies.

    b. produce antigens that attack the graft.

    c. cause elevations in white blood cell count.

    d. depress the immune system.

8. An adverse effect of immunosuppression is the development of

    a. chronic lung disease.

    b. lupus erythematosus.

    c. ascites.

    d. opportunistic infections.

9. Persons receiving azathioprine (Imuran) should be observed for adverse effects of the drug, including

    a. tachycardia.

    b. peripheral edema.

    c. drop in WBC.

    d. severe diarrhea.

10. K.C. is receiving immunosuppressive agents after a lung transplant. For which one of the following assessments would you contact the physician?

    a. Weight gain of 1.5 lb

    b. Temperature of 37.8°C

    c. Cough

    d. Hypoactive bowel sounds

■ Critical Thinking Case Study

M.B., a 12-year-old who received a kidney transplant yesterday, is taking cyclosporine (Sandimmune), azathioprine (Imuran), and prednisone to prevent rejection of the transplanted organ. (The learner may need to use additional sources to answer these questions.)

1. Identify what you will be assessing for, and your rationale for each assessment.

2. Describe the adverse effects of these medications.

3. Discuss the teaching that you will do regarding the medications M.B. is taking.

M.B.'s urinary output is minimal and her physician decides to dialyze her. M.B. starts crying, stating, "I've lost my kidney, haven't I?"

4. Describe the best response to M.B.'s statement.

Study Guide to Accompany Clinical Drug Therapy: Rationales for Nursing Practice, sixth edition, by Gail Ropelewski-Ryan.

CHAPTER 46

Physiology of the Respiratory System

■ Matching Exercise

TERMS AND CONCEPTS

Match the concept with the term for it.

1. _____ Hairlike projections that sweep mucus toward the pharynx.

2. _____ The functional units of the lungs.

3. _____ The lining adhering to the surface of the lung.

4. _____ The ability of the lungs to stretch or expand.

5. _____ Regulates the rate and depth of respiration.

6. _____ Stimulates the respiratory center.

7. _____ The normal percentage of oxygen contained in room air.

8. _____ Average tidal volume.

9. _____ Causes bronchodilation.

10. _____ Responsible for carrying O_2.

A. Oxygen level

B. Carbon dioxide

C. Visceral pleura

D. Cilia

E. Lobules

F. Medulla oblongata

G. Pons

H. 35%

I. 500 mL

J. 800 mL

K. Compliance

L. Sympathetic nervous system stimulation

M. 21%

N. White blood cells

O. Hemoglobin

■ Respiratory System Diagram

Match the letter of the descriptive statement with the corresponding body part in Figure 46-1.

A. Warms and humidifies the air.

B. Where air exchange takes place.

C. Connects the upper and lower respiratory tract.

D. The vocal cords are located here.

E. The walls contain smooth muscle controlled by the autonomic nervous system.

F. This muscle aids in respiration.

G. Mainstem bronchi.

2._____

3._____

4._____

5._____

6._____

7._____

_____ 1._____

FIGURE 46-1

Study Guide to Accompany Clinical Drug Therapy: Rationales for Nursing Practice, sixth edition, by Gail Ropelewski-Ryan.

■ Review Questions

1. Which of the following causes a decreased respiratory rate?
   a. Fever
   b. Exercise
   c. Pain
   d. Opioids

2. Which of the following factors has the most significant impact on diffusion in the lungs?
   a. Lung size
   b. Pressure differences between gases on each side of the membrane
   c. Adequate circulation
   d. The number and depth of respirations per minute

3. The average number of sighs per hour.
   a. 1–2
   b. 3–5
   c. 6–10
   d. 12–20

4. The passageway between the upper and lower respiratory tract.
   a. Trachea
   b. Bronchioles
   c. Alveoli
   d. Bronchi

5. Which is one of the common signs and symptoms of respiratory disorders?
   a. Fever
   b. Cyanosis
   c. Hypertension
   d. Cough

6. You would document the breathing pattern of a person with a respiratory rate of 30 as
   a. normopnea.
   b. tachypnea.
   c. bradypnea.
   d. apnea.

7. An average tidal volume is
   a. 100 mL.
   b. 250 mL.
   c. 500 mL.
   d. 1000 mL.

8. Which of the following transports O_2?
   a. Hemoglobin
   b. Albumin
   c. Leukocytes
   d. Lymphocytes

9. Which of the following is responsible for bronchoconstriction?
   a. Parasympathetic nervous system
   b. Sympathetic nervous system
   c. Medulla oblongata
   d. Cerebrum

10. Cilia
    a. filter air.
    b. secrete mucus.
    c. mobilize mucus.
    d. humidify incoming air.

CHAPTER 47

Bronchodilating and Other Antiasthmatic Drugs

■ Matching Exercise

Match the drugs with their effects.

1. _____ Bronchodilators that also have a mild diuretic effect.

2. _____ Reduce intracellular GMP, a bronchoconstricting substance.

3. _____ Reduce inflammation and mucus secretion.

4. _____ Stimulate receptors in bronchial smooth muscle to produce bronchodilation.

A. Adrenergics

B. Xanthines

C. Anticholinergics

D. Corticosteroids

■ Fill in the Blanks

Complete the following sentences.

1. Bronchoconstriction may be precipitated by

   a. _____.
   b. _____.
   c. _____.
   d. _____.
   e. _____.
   f. _____.
   g. _____.
   h. _____.

2. Epinephrine (_____) is injected subcutaneously for an _____. The therapeutic effects will be seen in about _____.

3. Albuterol (_____) can be administered _____ or by _____.

4. Ipratropium bromide (_____) improves pulmonary function within _____ minutes. The common adverse effects seen with this drug are

   _____, _____,
   _____, _____,
   _____, and _____.

5. Beclomethasone (_____) (_____) and triamcinolone (_____) are corticosteroids and are administered by _____.

6. Cromolyn (_____) is indicated for _____.

7. Early signs of hypoxia include _____,
   _____, _____,
   _____, and _____.

8. Mechanical measures for preventing retention of secretions include _____,
   _____, _____, and
   _____.

9. If you are administering two inhalers, a bronchodilator and a corticosteroid, the one you should give first is the _____.

10. After inhalation of a corticosteroid, the client should rinse his or her mouth. This will help prevent a _____.

■ True or False

1. _____ Children require a lower dose of theophylline.

2. _____ Cigarette smokers require a higher dose of theophylline than nonsmokers.

3. _____ The physician needs to know the body weight of the client before the correct dosage of theophylline can be determined.

4. _____ Theophylline can cause bradycardia.

5. _____ If an individual has heart failure, a higher dose of theophylline may be required.

6. _____ Long-term administration of cortico-steroids to a child can result in growth retardation.

■ Review Questions

1. Your client may need to have his or her dosage of theophylline decreased if he or she
   a. uses insulin.
   b. takes cimetidine (Tagamet).
   c. exercises strenuously.
   d. drinks large amounts of caffeine.

2. You know that your teaching has been successful if your client, who is using beclomethasone (Vanceril), states
   a. "I will limit my intake of caffeine."
   b. "I may gain weight as a result of taking this medication."
   c. "Nausea and vomiting are common adverse effects of this medication, so I will always take it with meals."
   d. "I will rinse my mouth after each use of my inhaler."

3. Which of the following statements by your client leads you to believe that she has understood the teaching you have done regarding cromolyn (Intal)?
   a. "If my weight increases, I will need to increase the amount of medication I am taking."
   b. "I can expect to have severe coughing after taking this medication."
   c. "I will need to use a nasal decongestant along with this medication."
   d. "If I do not obtain a therapeutic response from the drug in a month, my physician will discontinue it."

4. An expected outcome after the administration of bronchodilators is all of the following except
   a. decreased dyspnea.
   b. decreased respiratory rate.
   c. decreased anxiety.
   d. decreased secretions.

5. You should instruct a person started on an ipratropium bromide (Atrovent) inhaler about the common adverse effects of this medication, which include
   a. throat irritation.
   b. bradycardia.
   c. insomnia and anorexia.
   d. headache and gastrointestinal upset.

6. The physician orders ipratropium bromide (Atrovent), albuterol (Proventil), and beclomethasone (Vanceril) inhalers for Mr. P. t.i.d. You should
   a. question the order; three inhalers should not be given at one time.
   b. administer the bronchodilators first at 5-minute intervals followed by the steroid 5 minutes later.
   c. administer each inhaler at 1-hour intervals.
   d. administer each inhaler at 30-minute intervals.

7. Mrs. P. has a theophylline level drawn and it is 30 μg/mL. You know that this level is
   a. just below a therapeutic level.
   b. a therapeutic level.
   c. slightly above a therapeutic level.
   d. a toxic level.

8. Mr. H. was admitted to your unit 6 months ago weighing 158 lb. His medications at the time of the admission were Theo-Dur 300 mg t.i.d., digoxin 0.125 mg q.d., and furosemide (Lasix) 20 mg b.i.d. You weigh Mr. H. and discover that over the course of the past 6 months, he has lost 40 lb. What will you do next?
   a. Continue to administer the medications as ordered.
   b. Question the Theo-Dur dose as being too high.
   c. Question the Theo-Dur dose as being too low.
   d. Administer the Theo-Dur every other day.

9. Which of the following is a drug that decreases the effectiveness of bronchodilators?
   a. Phenelzine (Nardil)
   b. Erythromycin (E-Mycin)
   c. Propranolol (Inderal)
   d. Cimetidine (Tagamet)

10. When administering intravenous theophylline ethylenediamine (Aminophylline) to Mrs. G., the nurse should observe her closely for

   a. dysrhythmias.

   b. hypertension.

   c. apnea.

   d. depression.

■ Critical Thinking Case Study

Jenny, a 12-year-old girl, is admitted to the emergency room with an acute asthma attack. She has a 9-year history of asthma and is allergic to animal dander and grasses. She is not aware of any exposure that could have precipitated her attack, but the attack did occur during basketball practice. Jenny states that she had also been "fighting off a cold" for a week. Jenny takes albuterol (Proventil) and ipratropium bromide (Atrovent). The physician starts Jenny on zafirlukast (Accolate) and orders methylprednisolone (Solu-Medrol) IV push.

1. Identify what questions you would ask Jenny to elicit more assessment information.

2. Identify why the medications were ordered.

Jenny complains of palpitations.

3. Identify what you will say to Jenny and what nursing actions you will take.

Jenny complains of epigastric pain and her physician starts her on cimetidine (Tagamet).

4. Identify your nursing actions.

Study Guide to Accompany Clinical Drug Therapy: Rationales for Nursing Practice, sixth edition, by Gail Ropelewski-Ryan.

CHAPTER 48

Antihistamines

■ Matching Exercise

TERMS AND CONCEPTS

Match the concept with the term for it.

1. _____ The release of this chemical mediator produces bronchoconstriction.

2. _____ Used to prevent motion sickness.

3. _____ Over-the-counter medication for allergic rhinitis.

4. _____ Given parenterally for treatment of a hypersensitivity reaction.

5. _____ A very potent antihistamine that produces significant sedation.

6. _____ Dry mouth and drowsiness occur with this medication.

7. _____ Drug of choice for severe anaphylaxis.

8. _____ Has antihistamine, antiemetic, and sedative effects.

9. _____ A treatment for urticaria/angioedema.

10. _____ An adverse effect of the administration of some antihistamines.

11. _____ A newer antihistamine that can cause headaches.

12. _____ When antihistamines are administered for their antiemetic effect, you should see a decrease in this symptom.

A Promethazine hydrochloride (Phenergan)

B. Histamine

C. Dimenhydrinate (Dramamine)

D. Drowsiness

E. Diphenhydramine hydrochloride (Benadryl)

F. Cetirizine (Zyrtec)

G. Chlorpheniramine maleate (Chlor-Trimeton)

H. Epinephrine

I. Clemastine (Tavist)

J. Hydroxyzine (Vistaril)

K. Headache

L. Loratidine (Claritin)

M. Dizziness

N. Nausea and vomiting

■ Definitions

Define the following terms.

1. Anaphylaxis _____

_____

2. Serum sickness _____

_____

3. Hypersensitivity _____

_____

4. Anaphylactoid reaction_____

_____

■ Review Questions

1. Which of the following statements by Mrs. H. indicates successful teaching concerning promethazine hydrochloride (Phenergan)?

   a. "I can still have my after dinner drink."

   b. "I will eat a diet high in roughage while I am taking this medication."

   c. "I will be careful when driving; this medication could make me drowsy."

   d. "I can take this medication as frequently as I need it."

2. Phenothiazines should be used with caution in individuals who have

   a. seizure disorders.

   b. hypertension.

   c. diabetes mellitus.

   d. prostatic hypertrophy.

3. Which of the following conditions could contraindicate the further use of promethazine hydrochloride (Phenergan)?

   a. Anorexia

   b. Vomiting

   c. Nausea

   d. Photosensitivity

4. Antihistamines should be used with caution in persons with a history of

   a. hypertension.

   b. thyroid dysfunction.

   c. prostatic hypertrophy.

   d. diabetes mellitus.

5. Which of the following is an expected outcome after the administration of antihistamines for Parkinson's disease?

   a. Increased muscle strength

   b. Decreased rigidity

   c. Decreased deep tendon reflexes

   d. Increased coordination

6. Which of the following antihistamines is effective in treating pruritus?

   a. Diphenhydramine (Benadryl)

   b. Clemastine fumarate (Tavist)

   c. Hydroxyzine hydrochloride (Atarax)

   d. Cyproheptadine (Periactin)

7. Antihistamines are effective in treating which of the following allergic reactions?

   a. Pruritus

   b. Bronchoconstriction

   c. Tachycardia

   d. Hypotension

8. Which of the following antihistamines is effective in treating vertigo?

   a. Trimeprazine tartrate (Temaril)

   b. Methdilazine (Tacaryl)

   c. Cyclizine hydrochloride (Marezine hydrochloride)

   d. Meclizine hydrochloride (Antivert)

9. Which of the following is a newer antihistamine that does not cause drowsiness?

   a. Diphenhydramine (Benadryl)

   b. Diphenylpyraline hydrochloride (Hispril)

   c. Azatadine maleate (Optimine)

   d. Loratidine (Claritin)

10. What instructions should you give Mr. C., age 79, who is starting diphenhydramine hydrochloride (Benadryl)?

    a. "If your nose begins to run, use a nasal spray."

    b. "Constipation is common. Increase the roughage in your diet."

    c. "Decrease your sodium intake while you are using this medication."

    d. "Incontinence is an adverse effect of this medication. Contact your physician if it occurs."

■ Critical Thinking Case Study

Mrs. J. is a 55-year-old woman recently diagnosed with vertigo. The physician orders meclizine hydrochloride (Antivert). (The learner may need additional sources to answer the questions below.)

1. Discuss with Mrs. J. the reason the medication was ordered and the potential adverse effects.

Mrs. J. is very distressed about her diagnosis and asks you if there are any other medications that will help her.

2. Identify your response.

CHAPTER 49

Nasal Decongestants, Antitussives, Mucolytics, and Cold Remedies

■ Fill in the Blanks

Complete the following sentences.

1. Upper respiratory disorders include

   _____, _____,
   _____, _____, and
   _____.

2. Coryza is _____.

3. A prominent symptom of respiratory tract infection is a _____.

4. Nonrespiratory conditions that predispose individuals to secretion retention include

   _____, _____, and
   _____.

5. Antitussives are used when a nonproductive cough interferes with _____ and

   _____.

6. This mucolytic is also used for treatment of acetaminophen overdosage: _____
   (_____).

7. Ingredients used in cold remedies include

   _____, _____,
   _____, _____, and

   _____.

8. If nasal decongestants are overused, they can cause

   _____.

9. Nasal decongestants can _____
   heart rate and blood pressure.

10. Adverse effects associated with the use of opioid antitussives include _____,

    _____, _____,
    _____, _____,
    _____, and _____.

11. When MAO inhibitors are administered with dextromethorphan, there is an increased risk of

    _____ and _____.

12. Before instilling nasal decongestants, you should have the patient _____.

13. Nasal decongestants should be administered to infants _____.

14. After administering cough syrups, the patient should avoid eating or drinking for _____.

15. Individuals who require expectorants for congestion should be encouraged to drink
    _____ daily.

■ Crossword Puzzle

ACROSS

1. A nasal decongestant.
5. A non-opioid antitussive.
9. Many over-the-counter decongestants can decrease _____ discharge.

DOWN

2. A mucolytic.
3. An ingredient found in Dristan.
4. Inflammation of the mucous membrane of the nose.
5. An antihistamine and nasal decongestant.
6. A topical spray for nasal congestion.
7. A commonly used medication for colds and cough that contains guaifenesin.
8. Agents that suppress coughing by depressing the respiratory center.

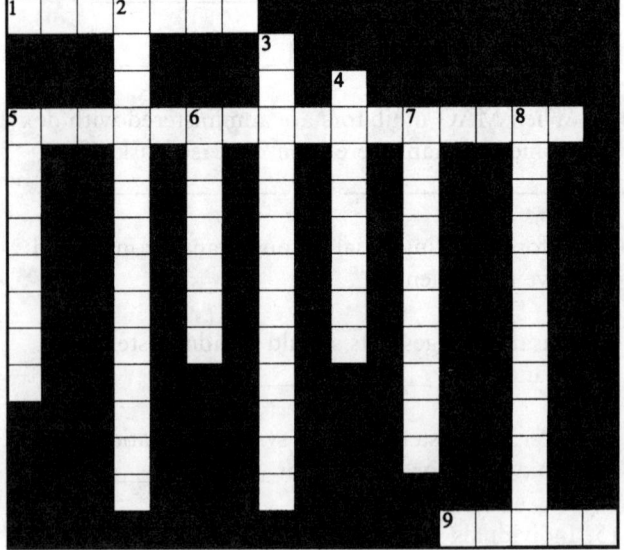

■ Review Questions

1. Which statement by your client would lead you to believe that he has understood the instructions you have given him regarding Mucomyst?
   a. "I will blow my nose before instilling the nasal spray."
   b. "I will report any dizziness, drowsiness, or rapid pulse."
   c. "I will drink 2000–3000 mL of fluid daily."
   d. "I will use it only when I am coughing."

2. An adverse reaction commonly experienced by persons using nasal decongestants excessively is
   a. diarrhea and vomiting.
   b. dry mouth.
   c. rash.
   d. rebound nasal congestion.

3. Which of the following statements by your client leads you to believe that he has understood the teaching you have done regarding his expectorant?
   a. "I should increase my intake of fluids."
   b. "It is best to take the medication with meals."
   c. "I should not drive while I am taking this medication."
   d. "I need to lie down for half an hour after I take this medication."

4. Which of the following groups of medications, if administered with decongestants, could increase their effects?
   a. Antianxiety agents
   b. Antihypertensives
   c. Anticholinergics
   d. Antihistamines

5. Which of the following medications could increase the risk of arrhythmias if administered with nasal decongestants?
   a. Antihistamines
   b. Thyroid preparations
   c. Theophylline
   d. Furosemide (Lasix)

6. Persons taking pseudoephedrine hydrochloride (Sudafed), a nasal decongestant, need to be observed for
   a. respiratory depression.
   b. constipation.
   c. tachycardia.
   d. muscle rigidity.

7. This medication is useful in treating an acetaminophen overdose.

   a. Acetylcysteine (Mucomyst)

   b. Tetrahydrozoline (Tyzine)

   c. Guaifenesin (Robitussin)

   d. Hydromorphone hydrochloride (Dilaudid)

8. An adverse effect of antitussives is excessive suppression of the cough reflex, which can cause

   a. apnea.

   b. tachypnea.

   c. retained secretions.

   d. increased pH of arterial blood.

9. A commonly used opioid in antitussive medications is

   a. morphine.

   b. Darvon.

   c. codeine.

   d. dextromethorphan.

■ Critical Thinking Case Study

Mr. Z., who has a 10-year history of COPD, has a temperature of 103°F. Congestion is audible upon auscultation, and his lung sounds are diminished in the bases bilaterally. The physician orders IV antibiotics, prednisone, guaifenesin, and acetylcysteine (Mucomyst). (The learner may need to use additional sources to answer these questions.)

1. Identify the instructions that you will give Mr. Z. before administering the medications.

2. Describe what you will be assessing for.

Mr. Z. has begun coughing up small amounts of tenacious sputum.

3. Identify your nursing actions.

Mr. Z. complains of being nauseated.

4. Identify your nursing actions.

5. Identify the instructions you will give Mr. Z. that may help prevent a recurrence of pneumonia.

CHAPTER 50

Physiology of the Cardiovascular System

■ Matching Exercise

TERMS AND CONCEPTS

Match the concept with the term for it.

1. _____ Membrane lining the heart chambers.

2. _____ The pacemaker of the heart.

3. _____ Responsible for increasing the heart rate.

4. _____ The smooth inner lining of an artery.

5. _____ Where the exchange of gases, nutrients, and waste products takes place.

6. _____ Helps maintain colloid osmotic pressure.

7. _____ Transports oxygen.

8. _____ Essential to blood coagulation.

9. _____ Functions as a defense mechanism against microorganisms.

10. _____ The resting or filling phase of the cardiac cycle.

A. SA node

B. Myocardium

C. Endocardium

D. Parasympathetic nerves

E. AV node

F. Sympathetic nerves

G. Intima

H. Leukocytes

I. Veins

J. Capillaries

K. Albumin

L. Hemoglobin

M. Diastole

N. Platelets

O. Systole

■ Fill in the Blanks

Fill in the blanks in Figure 50-1 with the terms below.

Aorta	Pulmonary artery	Left atrium	Left ventricle
Right atrium	Right ventricle	Superior vena cava	Inferior vena cava
Mitral valve	Tricuspid valve	Septum	Chordae tendon
Coronary arteries	Papillary muscle		

1. _____

2. _____

3. _____

4. _____

5. _____

6. _____

7. _____

8. _____

9. _____

10. _____

11. _____

12. _____

13. _____

14. _____

FIGURE 50-1

■ Review Questions

1. The portion of the heart that receives unoxygenated blood from the vena cava.
   a. Right atrium
   b. Right ventricle
   c. Left atrium
   d. Left ventricle

2. The valve that separates the right atrium and right ventricle.
   a. Mitral valve
   b. Tricuspid valve
   c. Pulmonic valve
   d. Aortic valve

3. The ventricles can beat independently at a rate of
   a. 10–20 beats per minute.
   b. 30–40 beats per minute.
   c. 50–60 beats per minute.
   d. 70–80 beats per minute.

4. These vessels carry lymphocytes and large molecules of protein and fat.
   a. Capillaries
   b. Lymphatic vessels
   c. Collateral circulation
   d. Arterioles

5. This plasma protein helps maintain colloid osmotic pressure.
   a. Fibrinogen
   b. Gamma globulin
   c. Leukocyte
   d. Albumin

6. This blood component is responsible for transporting oxygen.
   a. Reticulocytes
   b. Platelets
   c. Hemoglobin
   d. Leukocytes

7. Platelets are produced in the
   a. pancreas.
   b. adrenal glands.
   c. bone marrow.
   d. liver.

8. What percentage of plasma is water?
   a. 25%
   b. 50%
   c. 70%
   d. 90%

9. An increase in peripheral vascular resistance will
   a. increase blood pressure.
   b. decrease blood pressure.
   c. have no impact on blood pressure.
   d. make blood pressure harder to measure accurately.

10. Blood functions in all of the following ways except
    a. transporting oxygen to the cells and carbon dioxide from cells.
    b. carrying leukocytes and antibodies to sites of injury.
    c. producing components necessary for blood coagulation.
    d. regulating body temperature by transferring heat produced by cell metabolism to the skin.

CHAPTER 51

Drug Therapy of Heart Failure

■ Fill in the Blanks

Complete the following sentences.

1. When cardiac output falls, the body attempts to compensate by increasing sympathetic activity, which _____ the force of the contraction, _____ the heart rate, and causes _____. Aldosterone is released and causes increased reabsorption of sodium and water, which _____ blood volume and _____ blood pressure, resulting in _____.

2. As a result of these compensatory mechanisms, there is increased _____ and increased afterload.

3. Digitalis glycosides _____ myocardial contractility and allow the ventricles to _____.

4. Digoxin is used to treat atrial tachyarrhythmias, such as atrial _____ and atrial _____.

5. An oral digitalizing dose in an adult is _____ in 24 hours.

6. A child, age 2, weighing 22 lb, requires digitalization. The physician orders 0.04 mg/kg in four equal doses. How much medication will the child receive per dose? _____.

7. Kelly, a newborn who weighs 5 lb and has tetralogy of Fallot, is started on 0.025 mg/kg of digoxin. How much medication will the child receive per day? _____.

8. Amrinone (_____) can be used for _____ management of heart failure not controlled by digitalis and diuretic therapy.

9. Hypokalemia, hypomagnesemia, and hypercalcemia increase the risk of _____.

10. Factors contributing to digoxin toxicity are
    a. _____.
    b. _____.
    c. _____.
    d. _____.
    e. _____.
    f. _____.
    g. _____.
    h. _____.

11. Risk factors for heart failure include
    a. cardiovascular disorders
       1._____.
       2._____.
       3._____.
       4._____.
       5._____.
       6._____.
    b. noncardiovascular disorders
       1._____.
       2._____.
       3._____.
    c. other factors
       1._____.
       2._____.

12. For acute heart failure, the drugs of choice include _____, _____, and _____.

■ Matching Exercise

TERMS AND CONCEPTS

Match the concept with the term for it.

1. _____ A heart rate below 60.

2. _____ A complication of acute heart failure characterized by a buildup of secretions in the lungs and respiratory difficulty.

3. _____ The usual daily maintenance dose of digoxin.

4. _____ Administration of relatively large doses of digoxin.

5. _____ A drug used to treat digitalis-induced bradycardia.

6. _____ An electrolyte deviation that can increase the risk of digoxin toxicity.

7. _____ An arrhythmia in which the atrial heart rate is faster than the ventricular rate.

8. _____ An antidote for digitalis toxicity.

9. _____ A K-losing diuretic often used in the treatment of congestive heart failure.

10. _____ The route of digoxin administration used least often because it causes tissue irritation.

11. _____ A therapeutic digoxin level.

12. _____ A heart rate greater than 100.

13. _____ A nonpharmacologic treatment for heart failure.

14. _____ For chronic heart failure, ACE inhibitors are administered.

A. Digitalization

B. Orally

C. Sodium restriction

D. Digoxin immune fab (Digibind)

E. Atropine

F. Bradycardia

G. Hypercalcemia

H. Pulmonary edema

I. Intramuscular

J. Furosemide (Lasix)

K. 0.125–0.25 mg

L. 0.5–2.0 ng/mL

M. Atrial fibrillation

N. Tachycardia

■ Review Questions

1. When administering amrinone (Inocor), you should observe for the following adverse effect.

   a. Hyperglycemia

   b. Thrombocytopenia

   c. Hypertension

   d. Convulsions

2. An expected outcome associated with the administration of digoxin.

   a. Increased heart size

   b. Increased heart rate

   c. Decreased edema

   d. Decreased blood pressure

3. Persons taking digoxin and verapamil (Calan) concurrently may experience

   a. hyperglycemia.

   b. bradycardia.

   c. hypertension.

   d. convulsions.

4. A drug used for treatment of digoxin toxicity.

   a. Potassium chloride

   b. Propranolol (Inderal)

   c. Phentolamine (Regitine)

   d. Digoxin immune fab (Digibind)

5. When given with digoxin, which of the following medications will decrease the effect of digoxin?

   a. Isoproterenol (Isuprel)

   b. An antacid

   c. Furosemide (Lasix)

   d. Epinephrine (Adrenalin)

6. Your client is admitted with acute heart failure and is to be started on digoxin. Which of the following conditions would necessitate an alteration in the drug dose?

   a. Parkinson's disease

   b. Liver disease

   c. Impaired renal function

   d. Diabetes mellitus

7. Factors that predispose persons to digitalis toxicity include

    a. hyperthyroidism.

    b. hypernatremia, hypermagnesemia, and hypocalcemia.

    c. hypokalemia, hypomagnesemia, and hypercalcemia.

    d. concurrent use of phenytoin (Dilantin).

8. Mr. J. has a serum digoxin level drawn and it comes back 0.4 ng/mL. You know that this is

    a. below the therapeutic level.

    b. a therapeutic level.

    c. above the therapeutic level.

    d. a toxic level.

9. Mrs. P., who is taking digoxin (Lanoxin) 0.25 mg qd, furosemide (Lasix) 40 mg b.i.d., and potassium 20 mEq b.i.d., states, "What a lovely yellow blouse you are wearing this morning." Your blouse is white. What do you do?

    a. Evaluate Mrs. P. for other symptoms of digoxin toxicity.

    b. Withhold her furosemide (Lasix).

    c. Administer the medication as ordered. Mrs. P. is joking.

    d. Call her physician and ask for additional potassium supplement.

10. S.J. weighs 44 lb and is to be digitalized. The digitalizing dose is to be 0.03 mg/kg in three divided doses. How much will she receive per dose?

    a. 0.2 mg

    b. 0.3 mg

    c. 0.4 mg

    d. 0.6 mg

■ Critical Thinking Case Study

M., a 6-year-old girl weighing 42 lb, is admitted to your unit for treatment for heart failure. She is to be started on digoxin (Lanoxin), furosemide (Lasix), and potassium. The physician orders daily CBCs, digoxin levels, weights, and q4h vital signs.

1. Describe the digitalizing regimen to M.'s mother and tell her what she can expect.

2. Identify the adverse effects you plan to discuss with M.'s mother and why this information is important for her to know.

3. Describe the potential drug interactions you will discuss with M.'s mother.

M.'s mother asks why so many tests are being performed.

4. Explain the reason for the tests in terms both mother and child can understand.

6. Identify and prioritize three nursing diagnoses for a child with heart failure.

5. Identify ways of assessing compliance.

CHAPTER 52

Antiarrhythmic Drugs

■ Matching Exercise

TERMS AND CONCEPTS

Match the concept with the term for it.

1. _____ Irregular heart rate or rhythm.

2. _____ The heart's ability to generate an electrical impulse.

3. _____ Time during the cardiac cycle when the heart is unable to respond to a new stimulus.

4. _____ The normal pacemaker of the heart.

5. _____ An abnormal pacemaker.

6. _____ A life-threatening arrhythmia.

7. _____ Arrhythmias result from excessive.

8. _____ The ability of cardiac tissues to transmit electrical impulses.

9. _____ A prolonged PR interval.

10. _____ Symptoms of heart failure.

11. _____ These drugs are used to treat supraventricular and ventricular arrhythmias.

12. _____ Nonpharmacologic treatment for paroxysmal supraventricular tachycardia.

13. _____ A period of decreased excitability following contraction.

A. Automaticity

B. Arrhythmia or dysrhythmia

C. Fatigue and weight gain

D. First-degree heart block

E. Conductivity

F. Refractory period

G. SA node

H. Class IA

I. Sympathetic activity

J. Ectopic focus

K. Tachycardia

L. Carotid massage

M. Ventricular fibrillation

■ Crossword Puzzle

ACROSS

9. Drug used to treat atrial fibrillation.

10. Urinary retention can occur with administration of this drug.

DOWN

1. This medication should be administered with food to prevent GI upset.

2. Slows the ventricular rate; used with caution in heart failure.

3. This drug may be used to treat PVCs when lidocaine is ineffective.

4. For short-term treatment of ventricular arrhythmias.

5. May cause new arrhythmias or aggravate preexisting arrhythmias.

6. Used to treat bradycardia.

7. Rapid-acting drug given intravenously for supraventricular tachycardia.

8. Used to treat supraventricular tachycardia, atrial fibrillation, and atrial flutter.

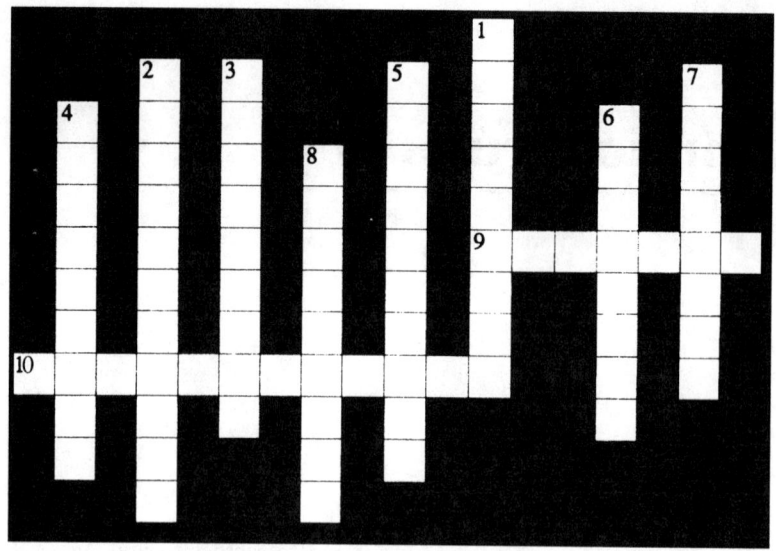

■ Cardiac Electrophysiology Exercise

PART I: DIAGRAM COMPLETION

Fill in the blanks in Figure 52-1 with the terms below to identify the components of the heart's conduction system.

Left ventricle   Left atrium   Right ventricle   Right atrium

Purkinje fibers   Bundle of His   Left bundle branch   Right bundle branch

SA node   AV node

10. _____   _____ 1.

9. _____

8. _____

7. _____

6. _____

5. _____

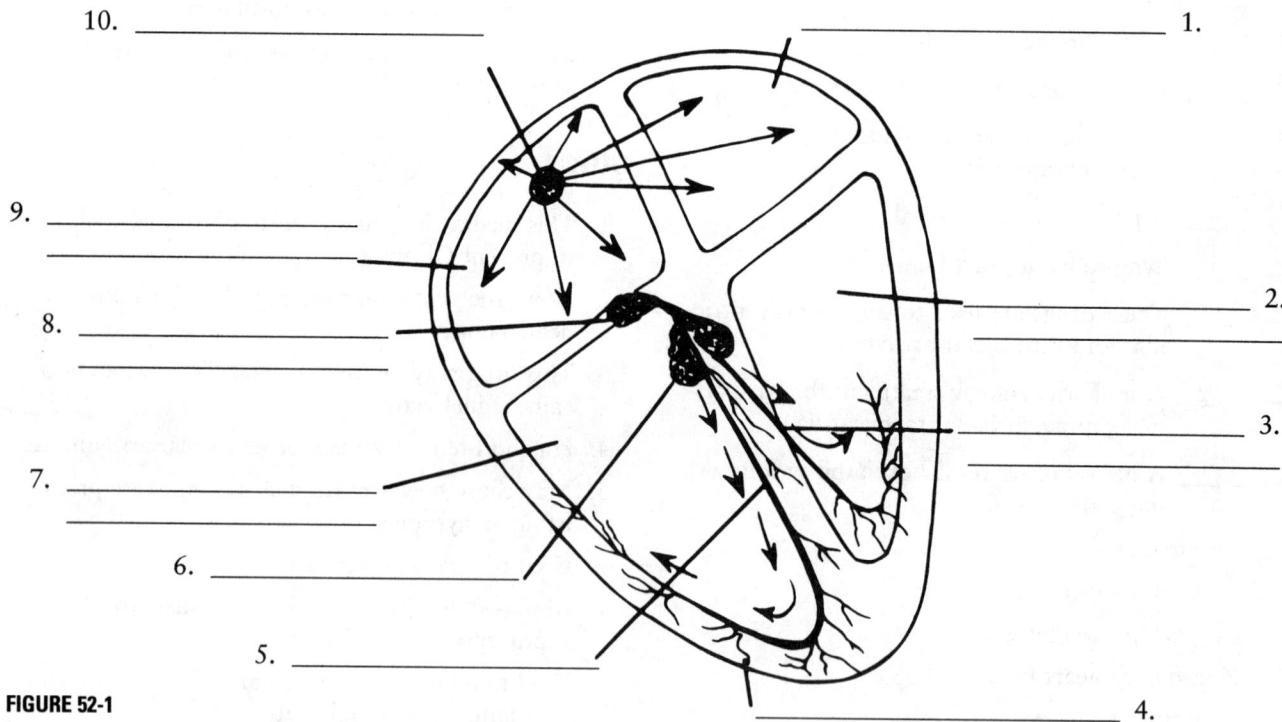

2. _____

3. _____

4. _____

FIGURE 52-1

PART II: DRUG EFFECTS ON CARDIAC PHYSIOLOGY

Use the numbers associated with the diagram from Part I of this exercise to complete the following sentences.

1. Pronestyl is used for treating serious refractory dysrhythmias originating in these heart chambers: _____ and _____.

2. Verapamil, a calcium channel blocker, is used to treat supraventricular tachycardia and atrial fibrillation and flutter because it slows conduction through the _____ and _____.

3. Atropine is the drug of choice for heart block because it improves conduction through the _____, and increases conduction through these parts of the heart:
_____, _____,
_____, _____, and
_____.

4. Disopyramide (Norpace), given orally to adults to treat ventricular tachyarrhythmias, works by reducing automaticity in the _____ node, slowing conduction through the _____ node, and prolonging the refractory period.

■ Dysrhythmia Analysis

Select the appropriate term from the list below to pair each of the dysrhythmias with a drug that might be ordered for its treatment.

Digoxin (Lanoxin)

Lidocaine (Xylocaine)

Supraventricular tachycardia

Adenosine (Adenocard)

Atrial fibrillation

Sinus bradycardia

Atropine

Premature ventricular contractions

1. Dysrhythmia _____ Treatment _____.

2. Dysrhythmia _____ Treatment _____.

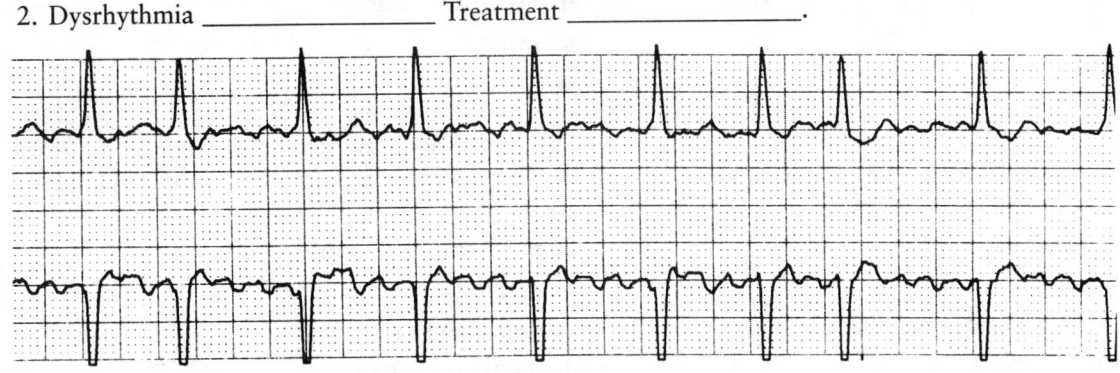

3. Dysrhythmia _____ Treatment _____.

4. Dysrhythmia _____ Treatment _____.

■ Review Questions

1. Which of the following conditions would require that the dosage of disopyramide (Norpace) be reduced?
   a. Seizure disorder
   b. Renal insufficiency
   c. Hepatotoxicity
   d. Diabetes mellitus

2. Side effects of amiodarone (Cordarone) therapy that the nurse should be observing for include
   a. hypotension.
   b. hallucinations.
   c. excessive bruising.
   d. cyanosis.

3. You find your client's IV drip of lidocaine running at 5 mg/minute. You know that this is
   a. below the therapeutic range.
   b. within the therapeutic range.
   c. above the therapeutic range.
   d. a highly toxic range.

4. Which of the following medications may be effective in treating PVCs that are refractory to lidocaine?
   a. Esmolol (Brevibloc)
   b. Bretylium (Bretylol)
   c. Verapamil (Calan)
   d. Adenosine (Adenocard)

5. Persons taking disopyramide (Norpace) should be observed for
   a. paralytic ileus.
   b. urinary retention.
   c. asthma.
   d. diarrhea.

6. The antidysrhythmic agent that is contraindicated for persons with severe uncompensated heart failure is
   a. phenytoin (Dilantin).
   b. quinidine.
   c. lidocaine (Xylocaine).
   d. digoxin (Lanoxin).

7. Your client asks you why he must take quinidine once he gets home. Your best response would be

   a. "Ventricular dysrhythmias can lead to the formation of thrombi on the atria."

   b. "Ventricular dysrhythmias will result in the ventricles beating independently."

   c. "Ventricular dysrhythmias may result in death."

   d. "Ventricular dysrhythmias can cause edema in your extremities."

8. An expected outcome after the administration of antidysrhythmia drugs is increased cardiac output, signs of which include

   a. no complaints of lethargy.

   b. adequate urinary output.

   c. a pulse rate above 80.

   d. no dyspnea.

9. Which of the following drugs, if administered with propranolol (Inderal), will decrease its effects?

   a. Atropine sulfate

   b. Furosemide (Lasix)

   c. Chloramphenicol (Chloromycetin)

   d. Digoxin (Lanoxin)

10. The physician has ordered 1 g of lidocaine (Xylocaine) in 500 mL D5W to run at 1 mg/minute. Using microdrip tubing, 1 mL = 60 gtt. How fast will you run the IV to deliver the correct amount of medication?

    a. 15 gtt/minute

    b. 30 gtt/minute

    c. 45 gtt/minute

    d. 60 gtt/minute

■ Critical Thinking Case Study

Mr. J., a 56-year-old man weighing 195 lb, is admitted to your unit with a diagnosis of myocardial infarction. You have standing orders in ICU that permit the use of lidocaine (Xylocaine) for treatment of six or more PVCs per minute.

1. Identify how much lidocaine you will administer as a bolus and how much you will use as a maintenance infusion.

Mr. J. continues to have multifocal PVCs that are uncontrolled by lidocaine.

2. Discuss alternatives to the present treatment and your nursing responsibilities.

Mr. J.'s PVCs have resolved, and you are preparing to send him to the cardiac catheterization lab. His ECG shows a P-R interval of 0.24 seconds. His heart rate is 60 and BP is 106/68.

3. It is time for Mr. J.'s propranolol (Inderal). In light of your observations, discuss what your actions will be.

Mr. J. is preparing for discharge. He expresses concerns about resuming an active sex life and asks if the Inderal will affect it. (The learner may need to use additional sources to answer this question).

4. Discuss your response to Mr. J.

CHAPTER 53

Antianginal Drugs

■ Fill in the Blanks

Complete the following sentences.

1. Nitrates work by reducing _____ and _____ and decreasing _____ and _____, which decreases _____ and _____. Nitrates increase blood _____ and lower _____.

2. Beta blockers reduce _____, _____, _____, _____, and _____.

3. A person receiving beta blockers should be observed for _____, _____, _____, and _____.

4. Calcium channel blockers dilate _____ and _____, decrease _____, and depress the conduction system.

5. Persons who have angina should avoid the following that could precipitate an attack: _____, _____, and _____.

6. Lifestyle changes that will help angina include _____, _____, and exercise.

7. Persons experiencing angina may take nitroglycerin, one every _____ minutes for a maximum of _____ doses. If the pain is unrelieved, they should _____.

8. Adverse effects from nitroglycerin include _____, _____, and _____.

9. Indicate adverse effects from administration of calcium channel blockers by placing an **x** next to the appropriate terms:

   a. _____ Heart failure.

   b. _____ Headache.

   c. _____ Diarrhea.

   d. _____ Weakness.

   e. _____ Anorexia.

   f. _____ Confusion.

   g. _____ Nausea.

   h. _____ Bradycardia.

10. If dizziness occurs after administration of antianginal drugs, the client should _____ and _____.

■ Matching Exercise

TERMS AND CONCEPTS

Match the concept with the term for it.

1. _____ A drug used for the long-term treatment of chronic stable angina.

2. _____ A calcium channel blocker used for angina and hypertension.

3. _____ A drug used for the treatment of supraventricular tachycardias.

4. _____ Onset of action of this drug is 1–3 minutes.

5. _____ A common adverse effect of antianginal drugs.

6. _____ This group of drugs used cautiously in persons with heart failure.

7. _____ A beta-adrenergic blocker given to prevent exercise-induced tachycardia.

8. _____ This group of drugs, when administered with antianginals, will decrease their effects.

9. _____ Tachycardia may occur with administration of this drug.

10. _____ This drug, when given with antianginal drugs, will increase their effects.

A. Nitroglycerin
B. Nicardipine (Cardene)
C. Anticholinergics
D. Hypertension
E. Isosorbide mononitrate (Imdur)
F. Nifedipine (Procardia)
G. Verapamil (Calan)
H. Beta-adrenergic blockers
I. Hypotension
J. Calcium channel blockers
K. Propranolol (Inderal)
L. Cimetidine (Tagamet)

■ Fill in the Blanks

EFFECTS OF NITROGLYCERIN

NITROGLYCERIN

1. Dilation of _____

2. Dilation of _____

3. ↓ _____

4. ↓ _____

5. ↓ _____

6. ↓ _____

7. ↓ _____

8. ↓ _____

■ Review Questions

1. The following complaint would indicate that Mr. J. is experiencing an adverse reaction to nifedipine (Procardia).
   a. "All of my joints ache."
   b. "I have been having severe headaches."
   c. "I have been having trouble breathing."
   d. "My ankles swell a lot, especially at the end of the day."

2. Which of the following instructions should you give your client, who is starting on nitroglycerin?
   a. "Once you get a headache, take no more medication because a therapeutic level has been reached."
   b. "You can take as much nitroglycerin as you need to control the pain."
   c. "If you become dizzy when you take the nitroglycerin, do not take any more."
   d. "You can take up to three tablets at 5-minute intervals. If you do not get relief go directly to the hospital."

3. Which of the following instructions should be included in the discharge teaching for a client discharged with a transdermal nitroglycerin patch?
   a. "Apply the patch to the front of the chest around the heart."
   b. "Apply the patch at the same time each day."
   c. "If you get a headache, apply the patch below your elbows or knees."
   d. "Apply a thin layer of cream to your skin before you apply the patch to avoid irritation."

4. A client, admitted with unstable angina, is started on a nitroglycerin patch and sublingual nitroglycerin. He asks you why both medications were ordered. Your best response would be
   a. "If your physician used only one medication, he would have to use a larger dose, which could cause you to have an adverse reaction."
   b. "The patch is for long-term prevention and the sublingual medication is for acute attacks."
   c. "It is very unusual for a physician to order two nitrates. I will speak to your physician."
   d. "If only a patch were used, such large doses would be required that skin irritation may result."

5. Your client has a history of alcohol abuse, hypertension, malnutrition, and asthma. What factors should the nurse take into consideration when a beta-adrenergic blocking agent is ordered for his angina?
   a. A person who ingests alcohol will require larger amounts of a beta-adrenergic blocker.
   b. Low serum albumin levels that result from malnutrition make it necessary to lower the dosage of beta-adrenergic blockers.
   c. Beta-adrenergic blockers are contraindicated for persons with asthma.
   d. Beta-adrenergic blockers may increase blood pressure.

6. Nitrates relieve angina pain by reducing afterload, which is
   a. blood volume within the heart.
   b. pressure within the heart.
   c. peripheral vascular resistance.
   d. oxygen demand of the heart.

7. Beta-adrenergic blocking agents help relieve angina by
   a. reducing oxygen demand of the heart.
   b. increasing the heart rate.
   c. increasing the blood pressure.
   d. reducing circulatory blood volume.

8. Your client is started on intravenous nitroglycerin. You should be observing him for
   a. hypotension.
   b. bronchospasm.
   c. congestive heart failure.
   d. ventricular arrhythmias.

9. Which of the following drugs, if administered with antianginal drugs, will decrease their effects?
   a. Promethazine (Phenergan)
   b. Digoxin (Lanoxin)
   c. Cimetidine (Tagamet)
   d. Isoproterenol (Isuprel)

10. Mrs. A. is taking atenolol (Tenormin) for angina, and you find that her pulse is 54. What should you do?

    a. Tell Mrs. A. to stop taking the medication and reassess her pulse the next day.

    b. Tell Mrs. A. to stop taking the medication and discuss it with her physician at her next appointment.

    c. Contact Mrs. A.'s physician and request that the medication be decreased.

    d. Instruct Mrs. A. to continue to take the medication as ordered.

■ Critical Thinking Case Study

Mr. D. comes to the emergency room complaining of severe chest pain. Three years ago his physician prescribed nadolol (Corgard) for hypertension, which he stopped taking last year because of sexual dysfunction. The physician starts a nitroglycerin drip.

1. Identify what assessments you will make during the infusion of the nitroglycerin.

Once Mr. D. has stabilized, he is started on diltiazem (Cardizem).

2. Explain the rationale for the choice of this drug to treat Mr. D.'s angina.

3. Identify the side effects of the drug that you will discuss with Mr. D.

Mr. D.'s physician also orders a nitroglycerin patch, which is to be put on at 6 AM and taken off at 10 PM.

4. Explain to the client why he is to use the patch in this way and what the potential side effects are.

CHAPTER 54

Drugs Used in Hypotension and Shock

■ True or False

1. _____ Alkalosis may decrease the effectiveness of dopamine (Intropin).

2. _____ Dobutamine (Dobutrex) will decrease cardiac output.

3. _____ When small doses of dopamine are administered, the client may experience hypotension.

4. _____ Epinephrine (Adrenalin) can produce ventricular arrhythmias and reduce renal blood flow.

5. _____ Isoproterenol (Isuprel) decreases the heart rate and increases diastolic blood pressure.

6. _____ If extravasation of dopamine (Intropin) or norepinephrine (Levophed) occurs, severe tissue damage can result.

7. _____ Dopamine (Intropin), dobutamine (Dobutrex), and isoproterenol (Isuprel) can be administered orally or parenterally.

8. _____ Vasopressors can increase oxygen consumption and produce myocardial ischemia.

9. _____ Beta-adrenergic blockers administered concurrently with vasopressors increase effects of the vasopressor agents.

10. _____ Adequate fluid therapy is necessary for dopamine (Intropin) to be effective.

■ Fill in the Blanks

Complete the following sentences.

1. Common symptoms of shock include _____ urinary output, _____ cardiac output, _____ orientation, seizures, cool extremities, and coma.

2. Drugs with alpha-adrenergic activity increase _____.

3. Drugs with beta-adrenergic activity increase _____ and _____.

4. When you are treating someone for shock, you want to keep their blood pressure above _____, their heart rate below 100, and their urinary output above _____.

5. The drug of choice for treating extravasation is _____ (_____).

6. The five types of shock are _____, _____, _____, _____ and _____.

■ Review Questions

1. Vasopressor drugs can increase oxygen consumption and cause
   a. postural hypotension.
   b. chest pain.
   c. confusion.
   d. abdominal distention.

2. This nursing diagnosis would take priority when caring for a client with anaphylactic shock.

    a. Altered tissue perfusion

    b. Altered comfort

    c. Risk for injury

    d. Altered bowel elimination

3. The doctor has ordered dopamine (Intropin) to treat your client's hypovolemic shock due to severe blood loss. For the medication to be effective, the physician must also order

    a. fluid replacement.

    b. beta-stimulating drugs.

    c. antibodies.

    d. fluid restriction.

4. An expected outcome after administration of vasopressor drugs is

    a. respiratory rate of 24.

    b. heart rate of 100.

    c. diastolic blood pressure between 80 and 100 mm Hg.

    d. urinary output of 30–50 mL/hour.

5. Mr. J. is started on an IV drip of isoproterenol (Isuprel) for hypotension after open heart surgery. What side effect will you be assessing for?

    a. Hypertension

    b. Tachycardia

    c. Dyspnea

    d. Cyanosis

6. J. has an IV hanging of 200 mg of dopamine (Intropin) in 250 mL of D5W (800 μg/1 mL). If the physician wants J. to receive 160 μg/minute, how fast will you run the IV (use microdrip tubing, 1 mL = 60 gtt)?

    a. 10 gtt/minute

    b. 12 gtt/minute

    c. 15 gtt/minute

    d. 18 gtt/minute

7. If you note that dopamine (Intropin) has extravasated, you should

    a. administer a beta-adrenergic blocker.

    b. apply a tourniquet.

    c. apply ice and elevate the extremity.

    d. administer phentolamine (Regitine).

8. Which of the following statements by Mr. P. leads you to believe that he has understood the teaching you have done regarding dopamine (Intropin)?

    a. "They will be adjusting this medication frequently to try and regulate my blood pressure."

    b. "I know that they will be monitoring my pulse frequently because it could drop."

    c. "This drug will increase the force of the contraction of my heart."

    d. "The doctor has ordered this medication to increase my heart rate."

9. Which of the following decreases the effectiveness of dopamine (Intropin)?

    a. Acidosis

    b. Alkalosis

    c. Hypokalemia

    d. Hypocalcemia

10. Beta-stimulating drugs should be used cautiously following a myocardial infarction because they can

    a. increase the peripheral resistance, causing decreased perfusion to the coronary arteries.

    b. decrease myocardial contractility and impair oxygen exchange.

    c. increase oxygen consumption and thereby extend the area of infarction.

    d. raise the blood pressure and therefore stress the heart.

■ Critical Thinking Case Study

Mr. B. is admitted to the ICU after an MI. He is presently experiencing cardiogenic shock. The physician orders dopamine 200 mg in 250 mL of D5W (Mr. B. weighs 220 lb).

1. Calculate the appropriate number of micrograms Mr. B. should be receiving per minute and identify the assessments that you will perform.

Study Guide to Accompany Clinical Drug Therapy: Rationales for Nursing Practice, sixth edition, by Gail Ropelewski-Ryan.

You have been unable to keep Mr. B.'s BP above 80/40, and his urinary output has dropped to 20 mL/hour. The physician decides to add dobutamine (Dobutrex).

2. Identify why Mr. B.'s physician is adding dobutamine (Dobutrex).

Mr. B. begins to experience chest pain. Nitroglycerin is added to his medication regimen. Mr. B. has standing orders for O$_2$ and morphine 2 mg. (The learner may want to use additional sources to answer this question.)

3. Identify why Mr. B. is experiencing chest pain, and list your nursing actions in order of priority.

CHAPTER 55

Antihypertensive Drugs

■ Matching Exercise

TERMS AND CONCEPTS

Match the drug group with its effect.

1. _____ Alpha$_1$ receptor blocking agents

2. _____ Alpha$_2$ receptor agonists

3. _____ Beta-adrenergic blocking agents

4. _____ Calcium channel blocking agents

5. _____ Diuretics

6. _____ Vasodilators

7. _____ ACE inhibitors

A. Block SNS impulses in the brain.

B. Decrease cardiac output and peripheral resistance.

C. Cause loss of sodium and water.

D. Cause dilation of blood vessels and decrease peripheral resistance; require concomitant use of a diuretic.

E. Dilate blood vessels and decrease peripheral resistance.

F. Decrease heart rate, force of contraction, cardiac output, and renin release.

G. Block the enzyme that converts angiotensin I to angiotensin II.

■ Name That Drug

1. _____ Used to treat acute childhood hypertension.

2. _____ A vasodilator that may be administered IM or IV for hypertensive crisis.

3. _____ Commonly used as an IV drip after open heart surgery to maintain the blood pressure within normal limits.

4. _____ A drug used for the treatment of mild hypertension that can cause potassium loss.

5. _____ These are the drugs of choice for persons over 50 with high renin levels.

6. _____ These drugs may be useful for persons who have angina and hypertension.

7. _____ This group of antihypertensive drugs stimulates the sympathetic nervous system, causing fluid retention.

8. _____ Available in a skin patch that can be applied once a week.

9. _____ A nonpharmacologic way of controlling blood pressure.

10. _____ These drugs are effective in treating hypertension for persons with renal disease.

11. _____ These antihypertensive medications produce hyperglycemia, hyperuricemia, and hypercalcemia in adults.

12. _____ Depression is an adverse effect of this medication.

13. _____ Abrupt withdrawal of this drug can cause a hypertensive crisis.

14. _____ ACE inhibitor used once daily for treatment of hypertension.

15. _____ Antihypertensive medications that are only used as step II or higher drugs.

16. _____ Insulin-dependent diabetic clients may have difficulty controlling their blood sugar if they are placed on this drug to control their blood pressure.

■ Fill in the Blanks

CARDIOVASCULAR INDICATIONS FOR USE

Place an x in the table to identify the appropriate indication(s) for each drug.

	Angina Pectoris	Hypertension	Arrhythmias	Heart Failure	MI
Losartan (Cozaar)					
Diltiazem (Cardizem)					
Nifedipine (Adalat, Procardia)					
Verapamil (Calan, Isoptin)					
Captopril (Capoten)					
Propranolol (Inderal)					
Metoprolol (Lopressor)					
Esmolol (Brevibloc)					

■ Review Questions

1. The physician prescribes captopril (Capoten) for Mr. B. You know that Mr. B. needs additional instruction regarding orthostatic hypotension if he says
   a. "If I become dizzy, I will eat something high in sodium."
   b. "I will make sure to rise slowly from a supine position."
   c. "I will not take hot baths and showers."
   d. "I will sleep with the head of my bed elevated."

2. Mrs. H., who is being treated for hypertension, should be instructed to avoid foods high in
   a. vitamin C.
   b. calcium.
   c. potassium.
   d. sodium.

3. Mrs. G. is admitted to the ICU complaining of chest pain. According to Mrs. G., her usual BP is 150/90. On admission, her BP was 170/100. Based on the latest readings, how would you classify Mrs. G.'s blood pressure?
   a. Mild hypertension.
   b. Moderate hypertension.
   c. Severe hypertension.
   d. Hypertensive crisis.

4. One effective group of antihypertensive drugs for treating hypertension related to high renin levels is
   a. ACE inhibitors.
   b. AIIRAs.
   c. calcium channel blockers.
   d. diuretics.

5. The physician orders nitroprusside (Nipride) 50 mg in 250 cc D5W to infuse at 1 μg/kg/min for Mr. J., who weighs 154 lb. How fast will you run the IV (using microdrip tubing, 1 cc = 60 gtt) to deliver the correct amount of medication?
   a. 21 gtt/minute.
   b. 23 gtt/minute.
   c. 25 gtt/minute.
   d. 27 gtt/minute.

6. The following lab value deviation is associated with the use of thiazide diuretics.
   a. Hypoglycemia.
   b. Hypernatremia.
   c. Hypocalcemia.
   d. Hyperuricemia.

7. The following instruction should be given to a client who is started on clonidine (Catapres).

    a. "Take the medication on an empty stomach."

    b. "Have your blood pressure checked daily."

    c. "Do not abruptly stop the medication."

    d. "Check your pulse before taking the medication."

8. For a person with a history of COPD who is experiencing hypertension, the selective beta-adrenergic blocker of choice is

    a. propranolol (Inderal).

    b. nadolol (Corgard).

    c. timolol (Blocadren).

    d. atenolol (Tenormin).

9. Which one of the following complaints may be directly related to reserpine (Serpasil)?

    a. Headache.

    b. Chest pain.

    c. Depression.

    d. Nausea.

10. The following medication may contribute to your client's elevated blood pressure.

    a. Tylenol.

    b. Synthroid.

    c. Oral contraceptives.

    d. Vitamin E.

■ Critical Thinking Case Study

Your client, M., is a 35-year-old female race car driver who weighs 200 lb and smokes two packages of cigarettes per day. Her doctor prescribes atenolol (Tenormin) for her essential hypertension.

1. Identify what lifestyle changes would help M. lower her blood pressure.

2. Identify why this medication was chosen for M.

3. Discuss the teaching you will do with M.

4. Identify ways of promoting compliance.

Three years after her initial treatment for hypertension, M. is seen at the physician's office. Her BP is 150/90 and she has symptoms of chronic renal failure. The physician changes her medication to enalapril (Vasotec) and bumetanide (Bumex).

5. Discuss why M.'s physician ordered two medications at this time.

Study Guide to Accompany Clinical Drug Therapy: Rationales for Nursing Practice, sixth edition, by Gail Ropelewski-Ryan.

CHAPTER 56

Diuretics

■ Fill in the Blanks

Complete the following sentences.

1. The nephron functions by three processes: _____, _____, and _____.

2. A minimum daily urine output of_____ is required to remove _____ of _____.

3. Most reabsorption occurs in the _____.

4. _____ promotes reabsorption of _____from the distal tubules and collecting ducts.

5. _____, a hormone from the adrenal cortex, promotes_____ reabsorption and _____ loss.

6. In the proximal tubules _____, _____, _____, and _____ are secreted.

7. In the distal tubules _____, _____, and _____ are secreted.

8. Edema occurs because of
   a. _____.
   b. _____.
   c. _____.

9. Diuretics are often used for persons with edema because they mobilize _____ by _____.

10. Diuretics are used for persons with hypertension because they decrease _____ and deplete _____, which may _____.

11. ____ are the most frequently prescribed diuretic agents. The diuretic effect occurs within _____ hours.

12. Potassium-sparing diuretics decrease the exchange of _____ for _____. _____ is the major adverse effect.

13. Osmotic agents increase _____ (_____), which causes _____ to be pulled from extravascular sites into the _____. _____ (Osmitrol) has many uses.

14. Before administering diuretics, the following blood values should be assessed because diuretics can alter these values: _____, _____, _____, _____, and _____.

15. Other assessments the nurse should do when a person is receiving a diuretic include measuring _____, _____, and _____, and assessing for _____.

16. When diuretics are given with digoxin, there is an increased risk of _____ related to _____.

17. A normal serum potassium level is _____.

18. If hypokalemia should occur, it can be treated in the following ways:
   a. _____.
   b. _____.
   c. _____.
   d. _____.
   e. _____.

19. Hypokalemia can produce the following symptoms:

    a. _____.

    b. _____.

    c. _____.

    d. _____.

    e. _____.

    f. _____.

    g. _____.

    h. _____.

    i. _____.

■ True or False

1. _____ Hypoglycemia is a common side effect associated with thiazide administration that can be reversed when diuretic therapy is discontinued.

2. _____ Hyperuricemia can cause gout in persons taking thiazide diuretics.

3. _____ Loop diuretics, when administered rapidly, can cause transient hearing loss.

4. _____ When loop diuretics are administered with aminoglycosides, the effects of the diuretic are decreased.

5. _____ Hypernatremia, hypermagnesemia, and hyperchloremia are common with the long-term use of diuretics.

6. _____ Loop diuretics and potassium-sparing diuretics should not be administered concurrently.

7. _____ The maximum daily dose of furosemide (Lasix) is 100 mg.

8. _____ Diuretics should not be administered to clients in renal failure.

9. _____ Nonsteroidal anti-inflammatory drugs can interfere with the effectiveness of diuretics.

10. _____ Diuretics should be started at a low dosage and gradually increased.

■ Fill in the Blank

THE NEPHRON

Fill in the blanks in Figure 56-1 with the terms below.

Descending limb of loop of Henle

Glomerulus

Ascending limb of loop of Henle

Loop of Henle

Efferent arteriole

Bowman's capsule

Afferent arteriole

Distal tubule

Collecting tubule

Proximal tubule

1. _____.

2. _____.

3. _____.

4. _____.

5. _____.

6. _____.

7. _____.

8. _____.

8. _____.

10. _____.

■ Review Questions

1. When loop diuretics are administered orally, you can expect to see a response to the medication in

    a. 5 minutes.

    b. 15–20 minutes.

    c. 30–60 minutes.

    d. 2 hours.

1._____

2._____

3._____

6. _____

8. _____

4. _____

5. _____

7. _____

9. _____

10. _____

FIGURE 56-1

2. Ms. H. is started on mannitol (Osmitrol) after an automobile accident to decrease her intracranial pressure. This drug works by

   a. promoting retention of sodium and water and excretion of potassium.

   b. blocking the exchange of sodium and potassium at the distal tubules.

   c. raising osmotic pressure, which pulls water from extravascular sites into the bloodstream.

   d. decreasing the reabsorption of chloride, bicarbonate, and sodium at the loop of Henle.

3. Edema is caused by decreased plasma osmotic pressure, which occurs as a result of the loss of

   a. capillary permeability.

   b. sodium.

   c. potassium.

   d. plasma proteins.

4. Which of the following is the most accurate way to assess a person taking diuretics for fluid retention?

   a. Weigh him daily.

   b. Measure his intake and output.

   c. Monitor his vital signs daily.

   d. Assess his electrolytes.

5. Which of the following lab values should be assessed to determine an adverse response to hydrochlorothiazide (Hydrodiuril)?

   a. Bicarbonate levels

   b. Glucose levels

   c. Calcium levels

   d. Chloride levels

6. Mr. C. has been using a thiazide diuretic for a year, and his serum potassium level is 3.1 mEq/L. This indicates that

   a. Mr. C. needs a potassium supplement.

   b. the dosage of the diuretic should be decreased.

   c. the dosage of the diuretic should be increased.

   d. the diuretic should be discontinued.

7. Identify why spironolactone (Aldactone) and furosemide (Lasix) are ordered together.

   a. Moderate doses of two different types of diuretics are more effective than a large dose of one type.

   b. This combination promotes diuresis but eliminates hypokalemia.

   c. This combination prevents dehydration and hypovolemia.

   d. Using two drugs increases osmolality of plasma and the glomerular filtration rate.

8. You will check the lab values of your client who has started on furosemide (Lasix) because you know a side effect of this medication is

   a. hyperchloremia.

   b. hypernatremia.

   c. hypokalemia.

   d. hypophosphatemia.

9. Which of the following is a loop diuretic?

   a. Spironolactone (Aldactone)

   b. Bumetanide (Bumex)

   c. Mannitol (Osmitrol)

   d. Hydrochlorothiazide (Hydrodiuril)

10. Your client is admitted to the hospital with pneumonia, and he has a history of chronic renal insufficiency. His physician orders furosemide (Lasix) 40 mg b.i.d. because it

   a. will not cause potassium loss.

   b. is effective in treating persons with pulmonary congestion.

   c. is effective in persons with renal insufficiency.

   d. will increase his PO_2 levels.

■ Critical Thinking Case Study

Mr. P., a 69-year-old man, is admitted with acute heart failure. His physician orders digoxin (Lanoxin) 0.25 mg q.d., furosemide (Lasix) 20 mg b.i.d., and spironolactone (Aldactone) 25 mg b.i.d.

1. Discuss why Mr. P.'s physician ordered these medications.

2. Identify what you should be assessing for (including lab values).

Three days after admission, Mr. P. has lost 10 lb. When you go into his room to do his morning assessment, you find that he is confused.

3. Identify your nursing actions.

CHAPTER 57

Drugs That Affect Blood Coagulation

■ Fill in the Blanks

DRUG INTERACTIONS

*Indicate whether the following drugs, when administered concurrently with Coumadin, will **increase** or **decrease** its effects.*

1. _____ Tetracycline.

2. _____ Aspirin.

3. _____ Dilantin.

4. _____ Maalox.

5. _____ Cimetidine.

6. _____ Estrogen.

7. _____ Inderal.

8. _____ Synthroid.

9. _____ Lasix.

10. _____ Phenobarbital.

■ Drug Indications and Actions

	Heparin	Coumadin	Retavase
1. Indications for use			
2. Onset			
3. Duration			
4. Route			
5. Blood tests			
6. Antidote			

▪ Review Questions

1. The effects of heparin are monitored by this lab test.

   a. CBC

   b. APTT

   c. PT

   d. BUN

2. Bleeding resulting from the administration of warfarin sodium (Coumadin) should be treated with

   a. Vitamin E.

   b. Vitamin K.

   c. protamine sulfate.

   d. calcium gluconate.

3. You know that Mr. J. has understood the teaching regarding anticoagulants if he states

   a. "I can still take over-the-counter medications if I have a cold."

   b. "I will inform my dentist about my medication before he performs any treatments."

   c. "I will use aspirin for arthritis pain."

   d. "I will continue to play rugby, but I will be careful."

4. Your client's PT is 20 seconds. This is

   a. a lower than therapeutic level.

   b. a higher than therapeutic level.

   c. a therapeutic level.

   d. a dangerously high level.

5. Your client is receiving heparin. After ABGs are drawn, you should hold his wrist

   a. 1 minute.

   b. 2 minutes.

   c. 4 minutes.

   d. 5 minutes or longer.

6. You know that Mr. C. needs additional teaching about Coumadin if he states

   a. "I will avoid walking barefoot."

   b. "I will not drink alcoholic beverages."

   c. "I will increase the dark green leafy vegetables in my diet."

   d. "I will contact my physician before I take over-the-counter medications."

7. Which of the following medications, if administered concurrently with warfarin sodium (Coumadin), will increase the risks of bleeding?

   a. Cholestyramine (Questran)

   b. Furosemide (Lasix)

   c. Cimetidine (Tagamet)

   d. Griseofulvin (Fulvicin)

8. You know that your client has a good understanding of why aspirin is being used if he states that aspirin will

   a. inhibit platelet aggregation.

   b. eliminate certain clotting factors.

   c. prevent blood from clotting.

   d. dissolve the clots.

9. Low–molecular-weight heparin (Lovenox) is administered in the

   a. abdomen.

   b. arm.

   c. love handles.

   d. leg.

10. The physician orders 18,000 U of heparin in 500 mL D5W to be administered over 24 hours. How many units of heparin will the client receive per hour?

    a. 575 U

    b. 650 U

    c. 790 U

    d. 825 U

▪ Critical Thinking Case Study

M., a 25-year-old woman, has been hospitalized with a fractured femur after a motor vehicle accident. M. weighs 200 lb, smokes one package of cigarettes per day, and is taking birth control pills and DiaBeta. M.'s BP is 180/90, pulse 90, and respirations 24 when she is admitted. During the night, she becomes short of breath and complains of chest pain. (Additional sources will be necessary to answer this question.)

1. Identify and prioritize your nursing actions.

The physician diagnoses M. with pulmonary embolism and starts her on a continuous infusion of heparin (1000 U/hr).

2. Discuss why M. was at high risk for developing pulmonary embolism.

M. is started on warfarin (Coumadin) while she is still receiving heparin.

3. Discuss why the two anticoagulants are being given together and identify how the dosage of Coumadin is determined.

CHAPTER 58

Drugs for Hyperlipidemia

■ Matching Exercise

TERMS AND CONCEPTS

Match the drug with its side effects.

1. _____ Cholestyramine (Questran).

2. _____ Gemfibrozil (Lopid).

3. _____ Lovastatin (Mevacor).

4. _____ Nicotinic acid (Niacin).

A. Flushing of head and neck.

B. Gastrointestinal discomfort, diarrhea, gallstones.

C. Constipation, flatulence.

D. Headache, skin rash, pruritus.

■ Fill in the Blanks

TREATMENT OF HYPERLIPIDEMIA

Treatment	Hyperlipidemia					
	I	IIa	IIb	III	IV	V
Cholestyramine (Questran)						
Pravastatin (Pravachol)						
Gemfibrozil (Lopid)						
Nicotinic acid (Niacin)						
Atorvastatin (Lipitor)						
Lovastatin (Mevacor)						
Diet modification						
Exercise						

■ Review Questions

1. Which of the following statements by your client leads you to believe that she understands the teaching you have done regarding cholestyramine (Questran)?
   a. "I will take the medication on an empty stomach."
   b. "I will increase the roughage in my diet."
   c. "I will weigh myself weekly."
   d. "I will have my blood pressure checked weekly."

2. Hyperlipoproteinemia is caused by this disorder.
   a. Alcoholism
   b. Diverticulosis
   c. Hypertension
   d. Hyperthyroidism

3. A drug that increases the effects of niacin is
   a. alcohol.
   b. insulin.
   c. prednisone.
   d. estrogen.

4. Once started on niacin, your client can expect to see a decrease in her cholesterol in
   a. 1 week.
   b. 3–5 weeks.
   c. 2–5 weeks.
   d. 1–3 months.

5. Flushing of the face and neck is a common side effect after administration of nicotinic acid (Niacin). Which of the following actions will decrease the flushing reaction?
   a. Administer niacin with an antacid.
   b. Administer aspirin 30 minutes before nicotinic acid.
   c. Administer diphenhydramine hydrochloride (Benadryl) with the niacin.
   d. Apply cold compresses to the head and neck.

6. A diabetic client, taking gemfibrozil (Lopid), should be told to report the following adverse reaction associated with the medication to his or her physician.
   a. Dizziness
   b. Headache
   c. Chest pain
   d. Diplopia

7. Which of the following statements by a client receiving an antilipemic leads you to believe that he or she needs additional teaching?
   a. "I will eat foods high in fiber."
   b. "I know I must lose weight and quit smoking."
   c. "I will exercise 20 minutes daily."
   d. "Now that I am taking this medication, I can eat whatever I want."

8. You should schedule a client receiving lovastatin (Mevacor) for the following tests because of the adverse effects associated with the medication.
   a. Monthly T_3 and T_3 levels
   b. Liver function studies every 4 to 6 weeks
   c. Monthly ECGs
   d. Weekly WBCs

9. Which of the following statements is true regarding antilipemics?
   a. Each drug is specific for one type of hyperlipidemia.
   b. All antilipemic drugs are effective against all types of hyperlipidemia.
   c. Each drug is recommended for specific types of hyperlipidemia.
   d. No antilipemic will also lower triglycerides.

10. Cholestryamine (Questran), a bile acid sequestering agent, can cause a deficiency in which of the following vitamins?
    a. Vitamin B_6
    b. Vitamin B_{12}
    c. Vitamin C
    d. Vitamin D

CHAPTER 59

Physiology of the Digestive System

■ Matching Exercise

TERMS AND CONCEPTS

Match the concept with the term for it.

1. _____ Propels food through the GI tract.

2. _____ Stimulation of this system increases motility and secretions.

3. _____ This system shunts blood away from the digestive tract.

4. _____ Muscular, fibrous tube whose main function is to convey food to the stomach.

5. _____ Secretes intrinsic factor.

6. _____ The sphincter at the beginning of the duodenum.

7. _____ When the stomach normally empties.

8. _____ A hormone produced by the duodenal mucosa that inhibits gastric secretion and motility.

9. _____ The first 10–12 inches of the small intestine.

10. _____ The portion of the small intestine that opens into the cecum.

11. _____ The portion of the intestine that absorbs water.

12. _____ This organ secretes enzymes that are necessary for digestion of carbohydrates, proteins, and fats.

13. _____ Releases bile when fats are present in the duodenum.

14. _____ This organ synthesizes bile, serum albumin, globulin, prothrombin, fibrinogen, blood coagulation factors, and urea.

15. _____ Provides the acid medium to promote pepsin activity.

A. Stomach
B. Enterogastrone
C. Duodenum
D. Peristalsis
E. Parasympathetic nervous system
F. Sympathetic nervous system
G. Esophagus
H. Trachea
I. Pyloric
J. Cardiac
K. 4 hours
L. 2 hours
M. Ileum
N. Colon
O. Pancreas
P. Gallbladder
Q. Liver
R. Hydrochloric acid
S. Bile
T. Gastrin

■ Digestive System Diagram

Match the organ with its function by filling in the blanks in Figure 59-1 with the letters below.

A. Absorption of most oral medications takes place here.

B. Water is absorbed here.

C. Secretes enzymes necessary for digestion.

D. Most drugs are metabolized here.

E. Releases bile when fats are present in the intestine.

F. Starch digestion starts here.

G. Protein breakdown occurs here.

1. _____ Stomach
2. _____ Pancreas
3. _____ Small intestine
4. _____ Large intestine
5. _____ Gallbladder
6. _____ Liver
7. _____ Buccal cavity

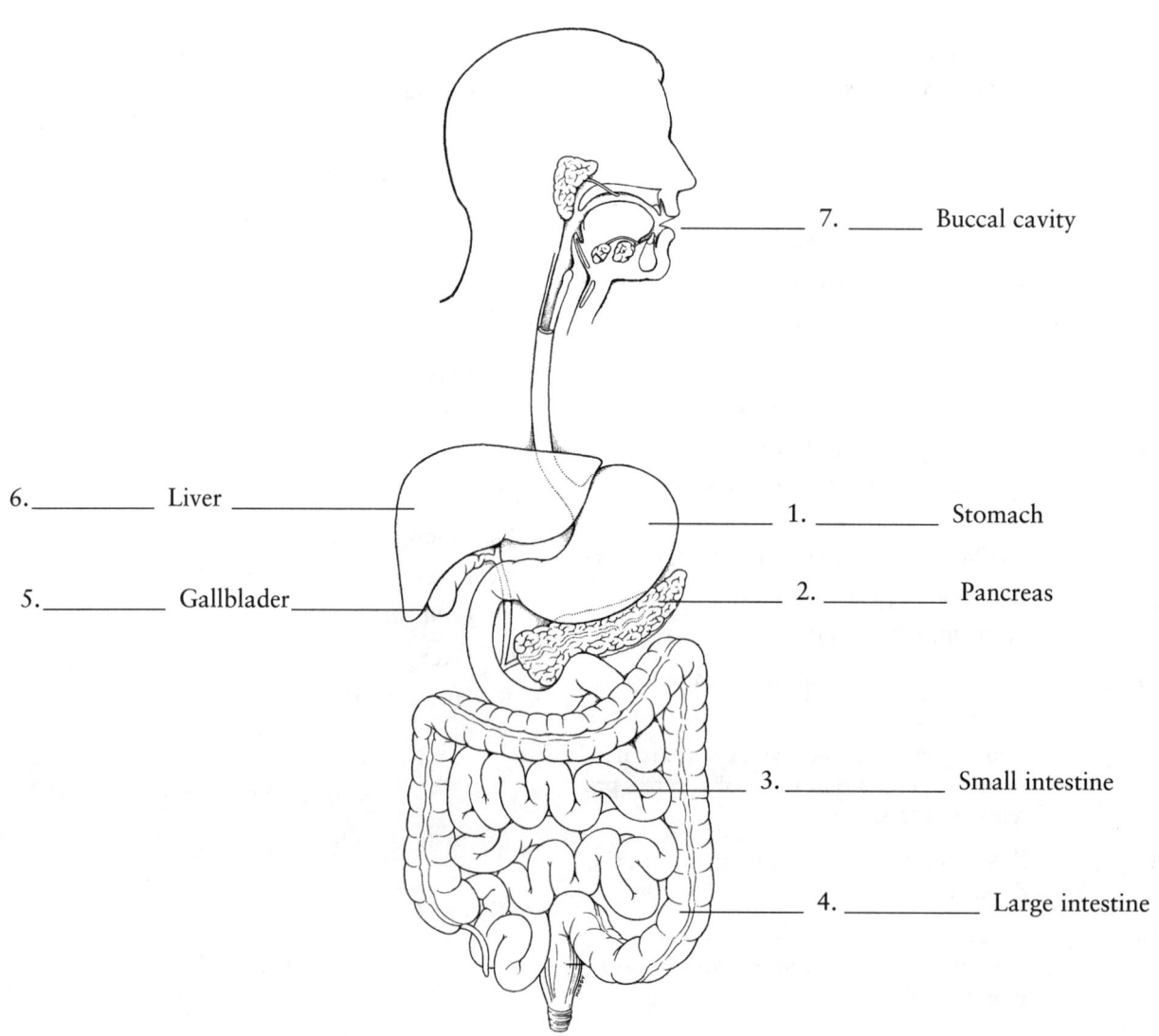

6. _____ Liver _____

5. _____ Gallbladder_____

7. _____ Buccal cavity

1. _____ Stomach

2. _____ Pancreas

3. _____ Small intestine

4. _____ Large intestine

FIGURE 59-1

■ Review Questions

1. When liver function is impaired, this substance can accumulate.
   a. Fat-soluble vitamins
   b. Hormones
   c. Glucose
   d. Cholesterol

2. Gastric juice has a pH of
   a. 1–3.
   b. 4–5.
   c. 6–7.
   d. 8 or above.

3. The major digestive enzyme in gastric juice is
   a. enterogastrone.
   b. gastrin.
   c. pepsin.
   d. lipase.

4. Bile is secreted by the
   a. gallbladder.
   b. liver.
   c. pancreas.
   d. small intestine.

5. The pancreas secretes all of the following, except
   a. amylase.
   b. lipase.
   c. cholesterol.
   d. trypsin.

6. The stomach empties in about
   a. 1 hour.
   b. 2 hours.
   c. 3 hours.
   d. 4 hours.

7. For the most part, digestion and absorption occur in the
   a. stomach.
   b. small intestine.
   c. large intestine.
   d. liver.

8. The liver breaks down worn-out erythrocytes and forms this waste product, which is excreted in bile.
   a. Bile salts
   b. Bilirubin
   c. Cholesterol
   d. Fatty acids

9. The body organ that produces 20% of the total body heat is the
   a. gallbladder.
   b. pancreas.
   c. liver.
   d. large intestine.

10. Blood flow to the GI tract increases with
    a. temperature extremes.
    b. pain.
    c. strenuous exercise.
    d. digestion.

CHAPTER 60

Drugs Used in Peptic Ulcer Disease

■ Matching Exercise

TERMS AND CONCEPTS

Match the concept with the term for it.

1. _____ Prevent the release of gastric acid into the stomach lumen.

2. _____ Inhibit gastric acid secretion.

3. _____ Increase mucus secretion.

4. _____ Slow onset and cause constipation.

5. _____ React with hydrochloric acid in the stomach to raise the pH (alkaline).

6. _____ May cause "acid rebound."

7. _____ Have a high neutralizing capacity, cause diarrhea and hypermagnesemia.

8. _____ Used to eradicate *H. pylori* organisms.

9. _____ Aluminum-based antacid used to lower serum phosphate levels.

10. _____ An antiflatulent.

A. Aluminum compounds

B. Gastric acid pump inhibitors

C. Histamine₂ receptor blocking agents

D. Prostaglandins

E. Antacids

F. Calcium compounds

G. Amphogel

H. Antimicrobials

I. Magnesium compounds

J. Simethicone (Mylicon)

■ True or False

1. _____ Alcohol and caffeine can cause gastric irritation.

2. _____ Protein and calcium in milk decrease secretion of gastric acid.

3. _____ Ulcers are usually treated with sucralfate (Carafate) for 2–4 weeks.

4. _____ Antacids increase the effectiveness of cimetidine (Tagamet) and sucralfate (Carafate).

5. _____ Avoiding highly spiced and gas-forming foods prevents ulcer formation.

6. _____ Stress stimulates gastric acid secretion.

7. _____ Omeprazole should be swallowed whole.

8. _____ Magnesium-containing antacids cause constipation.

9. _____ Proton pump inhibitors prevent the release of gastric acid.

10. _____ Histamine₂ receptor blockers decrease the acidity of the gastric juice.

■ Fill in the Blanks

Complete the following sentences.

1. Besides peptic ulcer disease, antacids are also used in the treatment of _____, _____, _____, _____, _____, and _____.

2. Omeprazole (Prilosec) inhibits the release of _____ into the stomach lumen.

3. H₂RAs decrease the _____, _____, and _____ of gastric juices.

4. Ranitidine (Zantac) is more _____ than cimetidine (Tagamet) and has fewer _____.

5. Famotidine (_____) and nizatidine (_____) are also used to treat ulcers but are less likely to cause _____ and _____ than cimetidine.

6. Misoprostol (_____) is indicated for clients with a high risk of _____.

7. Sucralfate (_____) adheres to the _____ and forms a protective_____ to promote _____.

8. Risk factors for peptic ulcer disease include
   a. _____.
   b. _____.
   c. _____.
   d. _____.
   e. _____.

■ Matching Exercise

The drugs below interact with cimetidine (Tagamet). Match them with their classification.

1. _____ Antiarrhythmics
2. _____ Anticoagulant
3. _____ Benzodiazepine antianxiety or hypnotic agents
4. _____ Beta-adrenergic blocking agents
5. _____ Bronchodilator
6. _____ Calcium channel blocker
7. _____ Tricyclic antidepressant
8. _____ Anticonvulsants

A. Carbamazepine, phenytoin
B. Verapamil
C. Alprazolam, chlordiazepoxide, diazepam, flurazepam, triazolam
D. Lidocaine, quinidine
E. Theophylline
F. Warfarin
G. Labetalol, metoprolol, propranolol
H. Amitriptyline

■ Crossword Puzzle

ACROSS

1. A synthetic form of prostaglandin E; helpful to counter gastric irritation caused by NSAIDs.

4. Antacids with high _____ content are contraindicated in edematous states.

9. _____ carbonate overuse may cause hypercalcemia.

10. Calcium antacids are rarely used for peptic ulcers because they cause _____ of gastric acid.

DOWN

2. This type of drug can cause abortion.

3. It is important that a patient be matched with an antacid that has this quality.

5. A drug that can prevent the development of stress ulcers.

6. Antacids containing this element may cause constipation.

7. A gastric acid-inhibiting drug administered once a day.

8. A cytoprotective drug that binds to ulcerated mucosa.

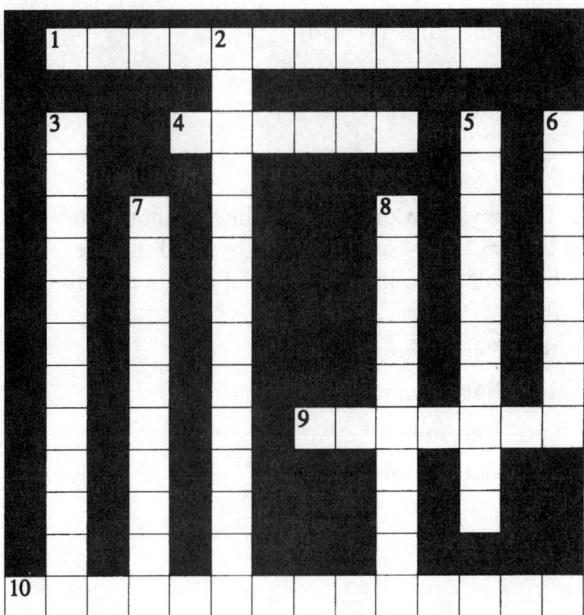

■ Review Questions

1. The ideal time to take antacids is
   a. 2 hours after meals.
   b. 1 hour before or after other drugs.
   c. ½ hour before meals with milk.
   d. with meals.

2. Your client is taking cimetidine (Tagamet). Which of the following statements would lead you to believe that he has understood the instructions?
   a. "I will take an antacid an hour before meals with the cimetidine (Tagamet)."
   b. "I will chew the tablets before swallowing them."
   c. "I will take cimetidine (Tagamet) with meals."
   d. "I will always take cimetidine with orange juice because it will enhance the absorption of the cimetidine."

3. Mr. J. has been treated for peptic ulcer disease with sucralfate (Carafate). His physician has recently added cimetidine (Tagamet). What adverse effect should you be observing for?
   a. Abdominal pain
   b. Nausea and vomiting
   c. Constipation
   d. Blurred vision

4. Which of the following medications is effective in preventing GI bleeding when administered with NSAIDs?
   a. Famotidine (Pepcid)
   b. Nizatidine (Axid)
   c. Misoprostol (Cytotec)
   d. Sucralfate (Carafate)

5. The physician orders ranitidine (Zantac) 50 mg in 100 mL D5W to be infused over 30 minutes. How fast will you run the IV (using macro gtt tubing, 1 mL = 10 gtt)?
   a. 27 gtt/minute
   b. 33 gtt/minute
   c. 42 gtt/minute
   d. 50 gtt/minute

6. Mrs. H., a 79-year-old woman with peptic ulcer disease, is taking cimetidine (Tagamet). When you enter her room, you find that she is confused. You should
   a. hold the medication until you have gotten her out of bed.
   b. hold the medication and contact her physician.
   c. stop the medication.
   d. administer the medication as ordered.

7. Persons taking aluminum compounds to neutralize stomach acid should be assessed for
   a. constipation.
   b. hyperphosphatemia.
   c. hypomagnesemia.
   d. diarrhea.

8. Mrs. H. is having a great deal of flatulence after her surgery. Which of the following antacids would be most helpful to her?
   a. Maalox
   b. Gelusil
   c. Titralac
   d. Aludrox

9. Magnesium-based antacids are contraindicated in
   a. hypertension.
   b. congestive heart failure.
   c. hepatic failure.
   d. renal failure.

10. Mrs. H. is in chronic end-stage renal failure. The physician prescribes Amphojel for her, to
    a. decrease her absorption of phosphates.
    b. increase her serum calcium.
    c. prevent gastric irritation.
    d. prevent constipation.

■ Critical Thinking Case Study

Mr. J. is admitted with gastrointestinal bleeding. His physician orders cimetidine (Tagamet).

1. Identify why Tagamet was ordered for Mr. J.

2. If 300 mg of Tagamet in 100 mL of D5W is to infuse over 20 minutes using macrodrip tubing (10 gtt = 1 mL), at how many drops per minute will you run the IV?

3. Identify the adverse reactions of the Tagamet you will be observing for.

Mr. J. is no longer bleeding and the physician orders sucralfate (Carafate).

4. Identify what you will be observing for.

5. Identify what foods should be avoided in peptic ulcer disease, and explain why.

6. Discuss the instructions you will give Mr. J. before discharge.

CHAPTER 61

Laxatives and Cathartics

■ Matching Exercise

TERMS AND CONCEPTS

Match the concept with the term for it.

1. _____ These substances swell and become gel-like and stimulate peristalsis and defecation.

2. _____ This laxative should be swallowed whole.

3. _____ These substances increase osmotic pressure in the intestinal lumen, causing water to be retained.

4. _____ These drugs irritate the GI mucosa, pulling water into the bowel lumen.

5. _____ Used as a suppository, it stimulates bowel evacuation by irritating the rectal mucosa.

6. _____ This lubricates the intestine by retarding colonic absorption of fecal water.

7. _____ A laxative that decreases the production of ammonia in the intestine.

8. _____ A substance commonly mixed with Kayexalate to prevent constipation.

9. _____ Used for fecal impaction.

10. _____ An adverse effect of the administration of mineral oil.

11. _____ Saline cathartics are contraindicated in renal disease because they may cause this.

12. _____ A product used to cleanse the bowel before surgery.

13. _____ This saline cathartic is less likely to produce hyponatremia because it has sodium sulfate as its major component.

14. _____ This laxative should be taken with a full glass of water.

15. _____ Discoloration of urine may occur with this laxative.

A. Saline cathartics
B. Mineral oil
C. Sorbitol
D. Stimulant cathartics
E. Bisacodyl tablets
F. Bulk-forming laxatives
G. Glycerin
H. Lactulose (Chronulac)
I. Oil retention enema
J. Decreased absorption of fat-soluble vitamins
K. Anemia
L. Hypermagnesemia
M. Hyponatremia
N. Magnesium citrate
O. Polyethylene glycol-electrolyte solution (GoLYTELY)
P. Cascara sagrada
Q. Psyllium preparations (Metamucil)

■ Definitions

Define the following terms.

1. Surfactant laxatives _____

_____.

2. Defecation _____

_____.

3. Constipation _____

_____.

■ Review Questions

1. Which of the following statements by Mrs. H. leads you to believe that she has understood how to use Metamucil?
   a. "I will drink the Metamucil as soon as I have it mixed."
   b. "I will mix the dry medication with apple-sauce."
   c. "I will use milk of magnesia in conjunction with this medication until I am having daily bowel movements."
   d. "I will decrease the roughage in my diet while I am using this medication."

2. Which of the following is a laxative used with Kayexalate to prevent constipation and aid in expulsion of the Kayexalate?
   a. Docusate sodium (Colace)
   b. Polyethylene glycol-electrolyte solution (GoLYTELY)
   c. Lactulose (Chronulac)
   d. Sorbitol

3. Mr. J. is to receive polyethylene glycol-electrolyte solution (GoLYTELY) for bowel cleansing before an endoscopic procedure. Which instructions should you give Mr. J.?
   a. "Take 1 gram every 4 hours followed by 8 ounces of fluid."
   b. "Take 1 ounce every hour until midnight."
   c. "Take 8 ounces every 10 minutes until the 4 liters are gone."
   d. "Take 1 ounce at bedtime and you will receive a cleansing enema in the morning."

4. An adverse effect of the administration of bulk-forming laxatives is
   a. impaction.
   b. vomiting.
   c. diarrhea.
   d. lower GI bleeding.

5. Administration of mineral oil can decrease the absorption of fat-soluble vitamins if continued for longer than
   a. 1 week.
   b. 2 weeks.
   c. 2 months.
   d. 6 months.

6. Long-term use of saline cathartics can produce this electrolyte imbalance.
   a. Hypermagnesemia
   b. Hypokalemia
   c. Hypochloremia
   d. Hyperphosphatemia

7. Medications that increase the effectiveness of laxatives when administered with them are
   a. anticholinergics.
   b. beta-adrenergic blockers.
   c. cholinergics.
   d. diuretics.

8. Before taking laxatives for constipation, Mrs. C. should
   a. drink 2000–3000 mL of fluid for several days.
   b. go to the bathroom every 2 hours.
   c. eat foods high in potassium.
   d. take a cleansing enema.

9. Mr. J. has recently suffered a myocardial infarction. Which of the following would be the most effective in preventing straining?
   a. Docusate sodium (Colace)
   b. Polyethylene glycol-electrolyte solution (GoLYTELY)
   c. Lactulose (Chronulac)
   d. Sorbitol

10. Which of the following laxatives acts by increasing osmotic pressure in the intestinal lumen and causing water to be retained?
    a. Lubricant laxatives
    b. Bulk-forming laxatives
    c. Magnesium citrate
    d. Stimulant cathartics

■ Critical Thinking Case Study

Mrs. J., a 79-year-old woman, has recently been admitted to your nursing home. She has had a problem with constipation for a number of years and is a chronic laxative user.

1. Identify nonmedicinal ways of dealing with constipation.

2. Discuss common causes of constipation.

Two days later, Mrs. J. still has not had a bowel movement. You contact the physician and he asks you what you think would work best for Mrs. J.

3. Identify your response and the rationale for your response.

CHAPTER 62

Antidiarrheals

■ True or False

1. _____ Very hot foods can cause diarrhea.

2. _____ Persons with a deficiency of lactase may have diarrhea when they eat dairy products.

3. _____ Severe diarrhea can result in metabolic acidosis.

4. _____ Diarrhea can be a symptom of stress in certain individuals.

5. _____ Hypothyroidism increases bowel motility.

6. _____ Chronic diarrhea can result in malnutrition and anemia.

7. _____ Psyllium preparations (Metamucil) are useful for both diarrhea and constipation.

8. _____ Withholding fluids is an effective way of treating diarrhea.

9. _____ Intestinal tumors can cause diarrhea.

10. _____ The drug of choice for treating diarrhea resulting from chronic inflammatory bowel disease is diphenoxylate with atropine sulfate (Lomotil).

11. _____ Cholestyramine (Questran) is the drug of choice for treating diarrhea due to bile salts.

12. _____ Loperamide (Imodium) is contraindicated for treating diarrhea due to bile salts.

13. _____ Side effects of diphenoxylate (Lomotil) include bradycardia and elevated blood sugar.

14. _____ Alcohol will decrease the effect of antidiarrheal drugs.

15. _____ You should report to a physician if your diarrhea persists for more than 3 days.

■ Fill in the Blanks

Complete the following sentences.

1. Causes of diarrhea include

   a. _____.

   b. _____

   c. _____

   d. _____

   e. _____.

   f. _____.

   g. _____.

   h. _____.

   i. _____.

   j. _____.

   k. _____.

2. Nonmedicinal approaches to diarrhea treatment include

   a. _____.

   b. _____

   c. _____

   d. _____

■ Review Questions

1. Which of the following medications is used to treat the diarrhea associated with pseudomembranous colitis?

   a. Lactobacillus

   b. Vancomycin (Vancocin)

   c. Pepto-Bismol

   d. Psyllium preparations (Metamucil)

2. Cholestyramine (Questran) is most effective in treating the diarrhea associated with
   a. Crohn's disease.
   b. bile salts.
   c. *Salmonella* infection.
   d. bacillary dysentery.

3. Which of the following medications, if administered with diphenoxylate with atropine sulfate (Lomotil), will increase its antidiarrheal effects?
   a. Antihistamines
   b. Cholinergic agents
   c. Thiazide diuretics
   d. Beta-adrenergic blockers

4. Which of the following statements by Mr. B. leads you to believe that he has understood the teaching you have done regarding loperamide (Imodium)?
   a. "It is not uncommon for there to be an increase in diarrhea initially."
   b. "I may experience dry mouth and urinary retention from this medication."
   c. "I should take the medication with foods high in potassium."
   d. "If I have a weight loss of more than 2 lb, I will contact my physician."

5. The nurse should assess for which of the following adverse reactions when administering colestipol (Colestid)?
   a. Nausea and vomiting
   b. Hypertension
   c. Constipation
   d. A papular rash

6. Which of the following antidiarrheal medications is used to treat diarrhea associated with ulcerative colitis?
   a. Cholestyramine (Questran)
   b. Psyllium preparations (Metamucil)
   c. Loperamide (Imodium)
   d. Sulfasalazine (Azulfidine)

7. Your neighbor calls you because she has been having diarrhea for 2 days. What advice should you give her?
   a. "Drink 2–3 liters of water every day."
   b. "Restrict your oral intake to decrease bowel stimulation."
   c. "Drink plenty of fluids that contain calories and electrolytes."
   d. "Eat dry crackers and cereal and only take sips of water."

8. Which of the following instructions should you give to your client who is taking cholestyramine (Questran) for diarrhea?
   a. "Always take the medication on an empty stomach."
   b. "Add at least 30 mL of water to each dose."
   c. "Do not take the medication within 4 hours of other medications."
   d. "If the medication does not control the diarrhea in 2 weeks, contact your physician."

9. Mr. J. has a history of diabetes mellitus, COPD, glaucoma, and hypothyroidism. For which of these disorders would the use of diphenoxylate with atropine sulfate (Lomotil) be contraindicated?
   a. Hypothyroidism
   b. Glaucoma
   c. COPD
   d. Diabetes mellitus

10. M.J., age 4, is admitted with an overdose of loperamide (Imodium). Which medication listed below is the antidote for Imodium?
    a. Lactulose (Chronulac)
    b. Diphenhydramine hydrochloride (Benadryl)
    c. Epinephrine
    d. Naloxone (Narcan)

■ Critical Thinking Case Study

You are a hospice nurse caring for Mr. N., who has an inoperable cancerous intestinal tumor and is receiving Sandostatin to help control his daily diarrhea. (The learner may need to use additional sources to answer the questions below.)

1. Identify the instructions you will give Mr. N.

The physician also orders Metamucil.

2. Specify the rationale for this order.

3. Identify the nursing assessments that you will make during each visit.

Mr. N. continues to have diarrhea and is having a significant amount of abdominal pain. His physician orders 2 mg of morphine q2h.

4. Discuss the nursing implications.

CHAPTER 63

Antiemetics

■ Matching Exercise

TERMS AND CONCEPTS

Match the concept with the term for it.

1. _____ A benzodiazepine useful in treating persons who experience anticipatory nausea and vomiting.

2. _____ A corticosteroid used for treatment of chemotherapy induced-nausea and vomiting.

3. _____ An anticholinergic used as a patch to treat motion sickness.

4. _____ Administered 30 minutes before chemotherapy to prevent/minimize nausea and vomiting.

5. _____ An over-the-counter medication administered orally at 15-minute intervals until vomiting stops.

6. _____ Used during surgical procedures to prevent nausea and vomiting.

7. _____ These drugs block the action of acetylcholine in the brain.

8. _____ These drugs block dopamine from receptor sites in the brain.

9. _____ The vomiting center is located here.

10. _____ Used as an antiemetic to prevent postoperative nausea and vomiting.

11. _____ A phenothiazine that acts on the CTZ and vomiting center.

12. _____ A cannabinoid used to manage nausea and vomiting during cancer treatment.

13. _____ An adverse effect of antiemetics.

14. _____ Vestibular branch of auditory nerve.

15. _____ Neurons in the fourth ventricle of the brain.

16. _____ Used to treat vertigo.

17. _____ A phenothiazine that can be administered rectally for nausea.

A. Dexamethasone (Decadron)
B. Granisetron (Kytril)
C. Phosphorated carbohydrate solution (Emetrol)
D. Antihistamines
E. Medulla oblongata
F. Dolasetron (Anzemet)
G. Phenothiazines
H. Droperidol (Inapsine)
I. Scopolamine (Transderm Scop)
J. Lorazepam (Ativan)
K. Promethazine (Phenergan)
L. Dronabinol (Marinol)
M. Concerned with equilibrium
N. Drowsiness
O. Prochlorperazine (Compazine)
P. Chemoreceptor trigger zone
Q. Meclizine (Antivert)

■ Review Questions

1. Antiemetics are usually contraindicated in clients with
   a. glaucoma.
   b. pregnancy.
   c. duodenal ulcers.
   d. angina.

2. The physician orders ondanestron (Zofran) for the management of Mrs. G.'s nausea and vomiting associated with her chemotherapy. Two days after starting the medication you find that Mrs. G. has a pulse rate of 108, a BP of 90/40, a macular rash, and a headache. Which of these symptoms may be related to the use of ondansetron (Zofran)?
   a. Tachycardia
   b. Hypotension
   c. Rash
   d. Headache

3. Persons using antiemetics may experience anticholinergic effects, which include
   a. dysphoria, drowsiness, and dizziness.
   b. dyskinesia, dystonia, and akathisia.
   c. dry mouth, blurred vision, and urinary retention.
   d. hypotension, confusion, and shuffling gait.

4. Which of the following statements by your client leads you to believe that she has understood the teaching you have done regarding prochlorperazine (Compazine)?
   a. "During episodes of nausea, I will drink clear liquids."
   b. "If I vomit, this medication can be administered rectally."
   c. "This medication should be taken on a full stomach."
   d. "I will need to decrease my sodium intake while I am on this medication."

5. The use of promethazine (Phenergan) is contraindicated in
   a. children under the age of 12 years.
   b. preoperative patients.
   c. pregnant women.
   d. persons under 100 lb.

6. Which of the following statements by your client leads you to believe that she needs additional instruction regarding antiemetics?
   a. "I will not drive while I am taking this medication."
   b. "Before I use any other medications I will contact my physician."
   c. "If I become drowsy, I will stop taking the medication."
   d. "If I experience adverse reactions to this medication, I will contact my physician."

7. Mrs. P. becomes nauseated the night before her chemotherapy treatments. Her physician believes that she is experiencing anticipatory nausea. Which of the following medications would be most effective for Mrs. P.'s nausea?
   a. Lorazepam (Ativan)
   b. Diphenhydramine (Benadryl)
   c. Hydroxyzine (Atarax)
   d. Trimethobenzamide (Tigan)

8. Mr. J. is going on an ocean cruise and is concerned about nausea and vomiting. His physician orders a scopolamine (Transderm Scop) patch. Which statement by Mr. J. leads you to believe that he understands how to use the patch?
   a. "I will put it on in the morning and take it off at night."
   b. "I will place the patch behind my ear and replace it every 3 days."
   c. "I will only use the patch if I feel nauseated or begin to vomit."
   d. "I will apply a thin layer of powder before I apply the patch to prevent irritation."

9. Mr. S. is receiving a phenothiazine for severe nausea. The nurse needs to assess Mr. S. for adverse effects, which include
   a. increased urinary output.
   b. hypotension and drowsiness.
   c. dizziness and depression.
   d. anorexia.

Study Guide to Accompany Clinical Drug Therapy: Rationales for Nursing Practice, sixth edition, by Gail Ropelewski-Ryan.

■ Critical Thinking Case Study

After radiation therapy, Mrs. B., who has a 10-year history of hypertension, experiences nausea and vomiting. Her physician orders lorazepam (Ativan).

1. Discuss why this medication was ordered.

2. Identify other measures that may be helpful in controlling nausea and vomiting.

Mrs. B.'s nausea and vomiting continue, so her physician adds prochlorperazine (Compazine).

3. Explain why this drug was chosen and the expected outcome after the drug is administered.

CHAPTER 64

Drugs Used in Oncologic Disorders

■ Matching Exercise

TERMS AND CONCEPTS

Match the antineoplastic agent with the disease process it is used for.

1. _____ Chronic granulocytic leukemia
2. _____ Hodgkin's disease
3. _____ Multiple myeloma
4. _____ Acute lymphoblastic leukemia in children
5. _____ Carcinoma of the breast
6. _____ Kaposi's sarcoma
7. _____ Bladder cancer
8. _____ Advanced endometrial carcinoma
9. _____ Rhabdomyosarcoma, Wilms' tumor
10. _____ Squamous cell carcinoma
11. _____ Palliation of ovarian cancer
12. _____ Cancer of the testes, bladder, ovaries
13. _____ Advanced breast cancer in post-menopausal women
14. _____ As an adjunct for palliation of symptoms in acute leukemia, Hodgkin's disease

A. Melphalan (Alkeran)
B. Methotrexate (Mexate)
C. Medroxyprogesterone (Depo-Provera)
D. Busulfan (Myleran)
E. Dactinomycin (Cosmegen)
F. Valrubicin (Valstar)
G. Daunorubicin (Daunoxome)
H. Fluorouracil (5-FU) (Adrucil)
I. Azathioprine (Imuran)
J. Cyclophosphamide (Cytoxan)
K. Carboplatin (Paraplatin)
L. Bleomycin (Blenoxane)
M. Tamoxifen (Nolvadex)
N. Prednisone (Meticorten)
O. Cisplatin (Platinol)

■ Fill in the Blanks

1. Most neoplasms are classified according to _____, _____ and _____.

2. They can also be broadly categorized as _____ or _____ neoplasms.

3. Leukemias and multiple myelomas are cancers of the _____.

4. Lymphomas are tumors of the _____.

5. Carcinomas are derived from _____ tissue including _____, _____, linings and coverings of_____.

6. Sarcomas are derived from _____ tissue including _____, _____, _____, _____ and _____.

7. Antineplastic drugs are classified as:

a. _____

b. _____

c. _____

d. _____

e. _____

f. _____

■ Cell Cycle

In spaces 1–5 provided in Figure 64-1, explain what happens during each phase of cell replication. On lines a–g, identify the antineoplastic agents that are effective in each phase.

Antibiotics

Alkylating agents

Podophyllotoxins

Nitrosureas

Antimetabolites

Steroids

Taxanes or taxoids

Vinca alkaloids

G_2

5. _____

_____

_____

h. _____

G_0

2. _____

S phase —

M phase

1. _____

a. _____

b. _____

4. _____

_____

_____

d. _____

e. _____

f. _____

g. _____

G_1

3. _____

_____

_____

c. _____

FIGURE 64-1

■ Review Questions

1. Your client has been started on busulfan (Myleran) for leukemia. Which of the following statements by your client leads you to believe that he has understood the teaching you have done?
   a. "If I have a fever or notice unusual bruising, I will call my doctor."
   b. "If I get short of breath, I will just rest."
   c. "Blood in the urine is common, so I won't be concerned."
   d. "I will call the doctor if I am nauseated."

2. Your client expresses concern that she will lose her hair during chemotherapy. Identify your best response.
   a. "Hair loss is temporary and reversible when the drug is stopped."
   b. "You may not lose your hair. Just wait and see what happens."
   c. "If you get a permanent wave, the hair that you have will appear thicker."
   d. "Some people lose their hair, but it grows back in nice and thick so don't worry."

3. Alkylating agents are more effective
   a. against resting cells.
   b. when there is organ impairment.
   c. when cancerous cells have metastasized.
   d. against dividing and resting cells.

4. An example of a hormone inhibitor used to treat breast cancer is
   a. ethinyl estradiol (Estinyl).
   b. medroxyprogesterone (Depo-Provera).
   c. tamoxifen (Nolvadex).
   d. cisplatin (Platinol).

5. You know that your teaching has been effective with a client receiving vincristine (Oncovin) if he states
   a. "I will avoid foods high in roughage."
   b. "I will drink plenty of fluids."
   c. "I will avoid foods that are high in iron."
   d. "I will weigh myself daily."

6. A priority goal for clients receiving chemotherapy is to
   a. accept their dying.
   b. remain free of infection.
   c. prevent bleeding.
   d. have a hematocrit above 35.

7. Your client, who is receiving chemotherapy for breast cancer, tells you that she has noticed ulcers in her mouth. The best response is:
   a. "Stay on a liquid diet until the ulcers have healed."
   b. "Your doctor can order a Carafate solution that will help the ulcers to heal."
   c. "Gargle with antiseptic solution after each meal to prevent infection."
   d. "Brush your teeth with baking soda and use a soft toothbrush."

8. When administering daunorubicin to Mr. H., the nurse should assess him for
   a. cardiotoxicity.
   b. pulmonary toxicity.
   c. neurotoxicity.
   d. renal toxicity.

9. You know your teaching has been effective if your client, who is receiving the hormonal antineoplastic agent prednisone (Deltasone), states, "I will take the medication
   a. on an empty stomach."
   b. about 1 hour after meals."
   c. with meals."
   d. at bedtime."

10. Alopecia is a common adverse effect associated with which of the following medications?
    a. Diethylstilbestrol (Stilbestrol)
    b. Megestrol (Megace)
    c. Medroxyprogesterone (Depo-Provera)
    d. Doxorubicin (Adriamycin)

■ Critical Thinking Case Study

Mrs. J. is receiving a combination chemotherapy regimen (FAC) of 5-fluorouracil, doxorubicin (Adriamycin), and cyclophosphamide (Cytoxan) for breast cancer.

1. Discuss with Mrs. J. why this regimen was chosen and what she can expect.

Mrs. J. begins to lose her hair, has developed stomatitis, and is extremely depressed.

2. Describe your nursing intervention.

Mrs. J. calls you to come quickly because there is blood in her urine. You examine the urine and find that it is red.

3. Discuss what your nursing actions will be.

One week after the initial treatment, you find that Mrs. J. has a respiratory rate of 28, a pulse of 102, and audible rales in her lung bases bilaterally.

4. Describe what you will do.

CHAPTER 65

Drugs Used in Ophthalmic Conditions

■ Matching Exercises

TERMS AND CONCEPTS

Match the concept with the term for it.

1. _____ May follow topical steroid therapy or injury.

2. _____ May be caused by inadequate lacrimation.

3. _____ A chronic infection in the lash follicles on the eyelid.

4. _____ Characterized by redness and watery discharge.

5. _____ Increased intraocular pressure.

6. _____ White, opaque, fibrous tissue that covers ⅚ of eyeball.

7. _____ The innermost layer of the eyeball.

8. _____ Constriction of the pupil.

9. _____ Dilation of the pupil.

10. _____ An elastic transparent structure that focuses light rays to form images on the retina.

11. _____ Produces a fluid that moistens and cleanses the eye.

12. _____ Light rays are deflected in various directions according to the density of ocular structures through which they pass.

13. _____ Nearsightedness.

14. _____ Farsightedness.

15. _____ Measurement of intraocular pressure.

A. Glaucoma
B. Conjunctivitis
C. Blepharitis
D. Keratitis
E. Corneal ulcer
F. Retina
G. Miosis
H. Lens
I. Mydriasis
J. Sclera
K. Tonometry
L. Hyperopia
M. Myopia
N. Refraction
O. Lacrimal system

■ Fill in the Blanks

Complete the following sentences.

1. Autonomic drugs are used preoperatively to _____.

2. Corticosteroids such as dexamethasone (Decadron Phosphate) are used to treat _____ of the eye.

3. A carbonic anhydrase inhibitor such as acetazolamide (Diamox) _____ intraocular pressure.

4. Fluorescein is a _____ used to _____ lesions or foreign bodies in the eye.

5. Cholinergic drugs used for _____ are instilled in the eye _____ times per day and cause the pupil to _____.

6. Anticholinergic drugs such as atropine are used before eye exams to _____ the pupil. Their use is usually contraindicated in the presence of _____.

7. Ocusert is replaced _____ and is used for long-term treatment of_____.

8. Two ocular effects of carbonic anhydrase inhibitors include _____ and _____.

9. Emergency treatment for chemical burns of the eyes includes _____.

10. The drug therapy for eye infections caused by the herpes simplex virus is _____ (_____).

■ Name That Drug

Identify the medications that cause the following adverse effects.

1. _____ Dehydration and hyperglycemia.

2. _____ Bradycardia and bronchoconstriction.

3. _____ Dry mouth and tachycardia.

4. _____ Nausea and paresthesias.

5. _____ Bronchospasms, heart failure, bradycardia, and hypotension.

■ Anatomy of the Eye

Fill in the diagram with the terms below:

Iris	Pupil	Scelera
Cornea	Anterior chamber	Optic nerve
Lens	Retina	Optic disc
Vitreous body	Choroid	

■ Drug Classification

Give an example of one drug in each classification and specify what it is used for.

	Medication	Use
1. Adrenergic		
2. Anti-adrenergic		
3. Cholinergic		
4. Anticholinesterase		
5. Anticholinergic		
6. Carbonic anhydrase inhibitor		
7. Osmotic agents		
8. Alpha$_2$ adrenergic agonist		
9. Anesthetics		
10. Lubricants		
11. Prostaglandin		

■ Review Questions

1. When administering eyedrops, you should
   a. not remove crusts around the eye before administering the medication.
   b. pull the lower lid down, drop the medication in the eye, and do not touch the eye with the applicator.
   c. pull the upper lid up and have the person look down; do not have them close their eyes for 1 minute after you have put the drops in.
   d. place one drop in each eye, wait 5 minutes, then place a second drop.

2. Your client is to go home on polyvinyl alcohol (Liquifilm). Your instructions should include the following.
   a. "Use one or two drops as often as you feel you need to."
   b. "Nausea, vomiting, and diarrhea are common side effects."
   c. "Lie down for 5 minutes after taking the medications."
   d. "If you experience blurred vision and photophobia, contact your physician."

3. Dipivefrin (Propine), an adrenergic drug, reduces intraocular pressure by
   a. contracting the sphincter muscle of the eye.
   b. preventing ciliary muscle spasm.
   c. decreasing production of aqueous humor.
   d. increasing outflow of aqueous humor.

4. Clients receiving demecarium bromide (Humorsol) will experience
   a. miosis.
   b. mydriasis.
   c. no pupillary change.
   d. double vision.

5. A person receiving anticholinesterase agents for a long period of time might experience side effects, including
   a. dehydration and hyperglycemia.
   b. corneal ulcerations.
   c. cataract formation.
   d. hypertension and dysrhythmias.

Study Guide to Accompany Clinical Drug Therapy: Rationales for Nursing Practice, sixth edition, by Gail Ropelewski-Ryan.

6. Which of the following statements indicates that the client understands the teaching you have done regarding pilocarpine (Pilocar)?

    a. "This drug can cause irritation and discomfort. My eyes may be red after I use these drops."

    b. "I know that I will have dry eyes, so I will use a lubricant after the pilocarpine."

    c. "The dosage of pilocarpine will need to be increased as I get older."

    d. "I can no longer drive an automobile."

7. Osmotic agents are used for

    a. treatment of chronic glaucoma.

    b. preoperative treatment for intraocular surgery.

    c. treatment of conjunctivitis.

    d. reduction of adhesion formation with uveitis.

8. The drug of choice for treating eye infections caused by a fungus is

    a. neomycin.

    b. trifluridine (Viroptic).

    c. Sulfapred.

    d. natamycin (Natacyn).

9. Pilocarpine is a miotic, which means it will cause

    a. dilation of the pupil.

    b. redness and swelling.

    c. burning and tearing.

    d. constriction of the pupil.

10. Medications that could elevate intraocular pressure include

    a. ibuprofen (Advil).

    b. meperidine (Demerol).

    c. prochlorperazine (Compazine).

    d. dexamethasone (Decadron).

■ Critical Thinking Case Study

Mrs. R. has come to the office for an eye exam because she had difficulty threading a needle. Her intraocular pressure is significantly elevated, so her physician orders timolol maleate (Timoptic) and pilocarpine (Pilocar).

1. Discuss why these medications were ordered for Mrs. R.

2. Identify the instructions that you will give Mrs. R.

Mrs. R. complains of burning when she instills the drops and asks you how long she will have to continue using them.

3. Discuss how you will respond to Mrs. R.

CHAPTER 66

Drugs Used in Dermatologic Conditions

■ Matching Exercise

TERMS AND CONCEPTS

Match the concept with the term for it.

1. _____ Pigment-producing cells.

2. _____ An inflammatory response of the skin to various injuries.

3. _____ "Hives."

4. _____ Chronic skin disorder characterized by dry, scaling lesions.

5. _____ Characterized by erythema, tenderness, and edema.

6. _____ An infection of the hair follicles.

7. _____ "Boils."

8. _____ A contagious skin infection.

9. _____ This fungal infection can occur following the use of broad-spectrum antibiotics.

10. _____ "Athlete's foot."

11. _____ A viral infection of the skin.

12. _____ Follicles become infected, and pustules, cysts, and abscesses are formed.

13. _____ A drying agent used for exudative lesions.

14. _____ An agent used to debride wounds.

15. _____ An agent used to remove warts, corns, or calluses.

16. _____ Fever blisters or cold sores on the lips.

17. _____ Inhibit growth of bacteria, viruses, or fungi.

18. _____ Shingles.

19. _____ Vitamin A derivatives used to combat acne, psoriasis, and wrinkles.

20. _____ A semi-solid preparation that adheres strongly to the area of application.

A. Dermatitis

B. Psoriasis

C. Folliculitis

D. Impetigo

E. Tinea pedis

F. Warts

G. Astringent

H. Enzyme

I. Acne vulgaris

J. Oral candidiasis

K. Furuncles

L. Cellulitis

M. Urticaria

N. Melanocytes

O. Keratolytic agent

P. Antiseptics

Q. Retinoids

R. Paste

S. Herpes zoster

T. Herpes simplex type I

■ Define

1. Macule _____

2. Papule _____

3. Nodule _____

4. Vesicle _____

5. Pustule _____

6. Erythema _____

■ Review Questions

1. The physician has ordered silver sulfadiazine (Silvadene) for your client's infected burn wound. She asks you why her physician has ordered this. The best reply would be:
   a. "This medication exerts antibacterial action against *Pseudomonas* organisms that infect wounds."
   b. "It is an excellent cleaning agent; it will dissolve necrotic materials."
   c. "Drug resistance can develop from other agents, so this medication is better."
   d. "When the skin is broken, more of the drug is absorbed systemically, so this preparation is more effective than oral agents."

2. An effective topical agent for psoriasis is
   a. calcipotriene (Dovonex).
   b. benzoyl peroxide.
   c. chlorhexidene (Hibiclens).
   d. pHisoHex.

3. Your client's physician prescribes triamcinolone acetonide (Aristocort) for dermatitis. An adverse effect of excessive administration of this medication is
   a. atrophy of the skin.
   b. superinfection.
   c. hypervitaminosis.
   d. increased pigmentation in the area of the application.

4. The physician orders acyclovir (Zovirax) for an initial outbreak of genital herpes. Which of these instructions should you give the client?
   a. "Apply topically to the lesions six times a day for 7 days."
   b. "Wash your perineal area before each application and use the medication in the morning and at bedtime."
   c. "You should leave the medication on for an hour, then remove it with soap and water."
   d. "Apply the medication no more than once a day. Overuse will cause severe inflammation."

5. The drug of choice for treating oral candidiasis is
   a. nystatin (Mycostatin).
   b. acetic acid.
   c. acrisorcin (Akrinol).
   d. zinc oxide.

6. The physician prescribes isotretinoin (Accutane) for severe cystic acne. An adverse effect of excessive administration of this medication is
   a. atrophy of the skin.
   b. superinfection.
   c. hypervitaminosis A.
   d. loss of pigmentation in the area of the application.

7. This agent is the drug of choice for treating warts.
   a. Salicylic acid
   b. Acetic acid
   c. Gentian violet
   d. Zinc oxide

8. Which of these medications would be most helpful to relieve itching associated with chicken pox?
   a. Coal tar (Balnetar)
   b. Colloidal oatmeal (Aveeno)
   c. Trioxsalen (Trisoralen)
   d. Sutilains (Travase)

9. Your neighbor calls you and asks you what ingredient would help her psoriasis. You should recommend a product containing
   a. benzoyl peroxide.
   b. hydrogen peroxide.
   c. coal tar.
   d. acetic acid.

10. Which of the following statements by Mr. R. leads you to believe that he has understood the teaching you have done regarding Retin-A?

   a. "I will apply the medication three times daily for 6 weeks."

   b. "My skin may become red and irritated from the medication."

   c. "I will soak my face in cold water before each application."

   d. "This medication will increase my tolerance to sunlight."

■ Critical Thinking Case Study

M., a 19-year-old college student, comes to the clinic to be treated for acne. She was previously treated at age 16 with tetracycline, with limited success. The physician starts her on tretinoin (Retin-A).

1. Identify what instructions you will give M.

M. returns 1 month later. Her facial acne is worse. She states that she has started taking birth control pills.

2. Identify the teaching that you will do with M.

Three months after she has received the medication, M. returns. Her face is excoriated and draining clear serous fluid.

3. Identify what you will do.

Study Guide to Accompany Clinical Drug Therapy: Rationales for Nursing Practice, sixth edition, by Gail Ropelewski-Ryan.

CHAPTER 67

Drug Use During Pregnancy and Lactation

■ Checklist

CONTRAINDICATED DRUGS

Place an x next to the drugs that should be avoided during pregnancy.

1. _____ Captopril (Capoten).

2. _____ Thiazide diuretics.

3. _____ Penicillins.

4. _____ Aminoglycosides.

5. _____ Tetracyclines.

6. _____ Corticosteroids.

7. _____ Laxatives.

8. _____ Oral antidiabetic agents.

9. _____ Quinidine (Quinaglute).

10. _____ Antimanic agents.

11. _____ Alcohol.

12. _____ Nicotine.

13. _____ Caffeine.

■ Matching Exercise

DRUGS AND INDICATIONS

Identify the medications that fit the following descriptions.

1. _____ Stimulate uterine contraction; used to initiate the birth process.

2. _____ Causes relaxation of uterine smooth muscle.

3. _____ Used to stimulate labor when uterine contractions are weak and ineffective.

4. _____ The drug of choice for treating pain during labor.

5. _____ Used after delivery of the baby if bleeding is severe.

6. _____ Administered to prevent asthma attacks.

7. _____ Used to treat anemia of pregnancy.

8. _____ The drug of choice for constipation during pregnancy.

9. _____ Used to treat hypertension associated with pregnancy.

10. _____ Intravenous medication that prevents seizures in preeclamptic mothers.

A. Terbutaline (Brethine)

B. Meperidine (Demerol)

C. Methylergonovine (Methergine)

D. Albuterol (Proventil)

E. Oxytocin (Pitocin)

F. Prostaglandins

G. Morphine

H. Magnesium sulfate

I. Apresoline

J. Metamucil

K. Ferrous sulfate

■ Fill in the Blanks

VASCULAR SYSTEM

1. Cardiac output _____
   30%–40% above the nonpregnant level at approximately the 24th week of gestation.

2. A _____% _____ in circulating blood volume occurs because an
   _____ in plasma renin levels stimulates the secretion of aldosterone, causing retention of Na^+ and H_2O.

3. Water-soluble drugs are more widely distributed, therefore drug dosage requirements may need to be _____.

4. Physiologic _____ develops because of hemodilution of the blood volume.

5. Decreased peripheral resistance results in dilation of the arterial system, causing pooling of blood. Therefore, BP does not go up even though there is a substantial _____ in blood volume.

6. Serum albumin levels _____;
   therefore, there is a _____ capacity for drug binding.

7. _____ glomerular filtration rate (GFR): up to 50% increase to clear creatinine, urea, and uric acid more quickly.

8. In early pregnancy there is _____ excretion of drugs by the kidneys. In late pregnancy there is _____ renal blood flow and _____ excretion and _____ effect of renally excreted drugs.

■ Review Questions

1. Mrs. S. is 6 months pregnant, and her physician tries to stop her labor with ritodrine (Yutopar). Which of the following maternal assessments will you do on an ongoing basis?
   a. Lung sounds
   b. Hourly urinary outputs
   c. Deep tendon reflexes
   d. Level of consciousness

2. An adverse effect associated with the administration of large doses of oxytocin (Pitocin) is
   a. respiratory distress.
   b. chest pain.
   c. convulsions.
   d. hyperglycemia.

3. The physician orders 4 g of magnesium sulfate in 250 mL of D5W to infuse over 4 hours. If you administer 1 g per hour, how fast will you run the IV?
   a. 63 mL/hr
   b. 78 mL/hr
   c. 82 mL/hr
   d. 100 mL/hr

4. Mrs. B. has epilepsy and is taking phenytoin (Dilantin) and phenobarbital. She is presently 4 weeks pregnant and she is concerned about the effect of the medications on the baby. Identify your response.
   a. "You have nothing to worry about. You are in the hands of a very competent doctor."
   b. "The doctor will probably discontinue your medications until you deliver."
   c. "You should abort this fetus because the medications have already done irreversible damage."
   d. "Maternal ingestion of these drugs may cause neonatal bleeding during the first 24 hours after birth. The baby will receive vitamin K immediately after birth."

5. Mrs. B. is 2 months pregnant and is complaining of nausea. Which of the following instructions will you give her?
   a. "Ask your doctor for an antiemetic."
   b. "Try dry crackers upon awakening. Usually the nausea goes away; if it doesn't, let your physician know."
   c. "Antacids will help; take them as often as you like."
   d. "Constipation makes nausea worse. Mineral oil is very effective in preventing constipation."

6. Mrs. C. develops pneumonia during her pregnancy. Which of the following antibiotics is the safest for use during pregnancy?
   a. Erythromycin
   b. Aminoglycoside
   c. Tetracycline
   d. Sulfonamide

Study Guide to Accompany Clinical Drug Therapy: Rationales for Nursing Practice, sixth edition, by Gail Ropelewski-Ryan.

7. Mrs. R. has been taking amitriptyline (Elavil) for depression and asks you about becoming pregnant. The best response to Mrs. G.'s inquiry is

   a. "There have been reports of congenital malformations and neonatal withdrawal when pregnant women take this drug."

   b. "You can use this drug if you discontinue it 1 month before delivery."

   c. "I recommend that you do not become pregnant."

   d. "There are studies that show growth retardation after birth in infants of mothers who take this drug during pregnancy."

8. Which of the following antihypertensive drugs is commonly used during pregnancy and is considered safe?

   a. Hydralazine (Apresoline)

   b. Guanabenz (Wytensin)

   c. Captopril (Capoten)

   d. Clonidine (Catapres)

9. Mrs. B. is receiving a magnesium sulfate drip. Which of the following assessments would indicate toxicity?

   a. Absence of deep tendon reflexes

   b. A 40-point drop in blood pressure

   c. Respiratory rate of 36

   d. Urinary output of greater than 400 mL in 1 hour

10. You prepare an IV of 1000 mL D5W with 10 U of oxytocin. The drip is started at 2 milliunits per minute. The physician's order is to increase the oxytocin 1 mU every 20 minutes. If you are using microdrip tubing (60 drops = 1 mL), by how many drops will you increase the rate of the infusion every 20 minutes?

    a. 2 drops

    b. 6 drops

    c. 10 drops

    d. 12 drops

■ Critical Thinking Case Study

Mrs. J. is brought to the hospital. She has been leaking amniotic fluid for 2 days, and her physician has decided to induce her. He orders a prostaglandin vaginal suppository, to be followed by an oxytocin (Pitocin) drip. Mrs. J. is extremely apprehensive and asks why she must receive these medications.

1. Describe how you will respond to Mrs. J.

Two hours after the initiation of the oxytocin drip, Mrs. J. complains of severe pain.

2. Identify what your nursing actions will be.

The physician orders meperidine (Demerol) IV push. During administration of the analgesic, Mrs. J. states that everything is going black and she appears to faint.

3. Identify and prioritize your nursing actions.

Comprehensive Critical Thinking Exercises

■ Thrombolytic Agents: Critical Thinking Case Study

S.K., a 34-year-old mother of four, is admitted to your unit with thrombophlebitis of the left leg. Her leg is swollen and tender from toes to mid thigh. She is also complaining of nonradiating chest pain. She is obese at 5'3" and 185 lb, and has a history of rheumatic heart disease. She takes birth control pills and DiaBeta. She has an elevated white blood count and sedimentation rate. Her temperature is 38°C and her pulse is irregular at 110. She is started on heparin, 20,000 U/1000 mL D5W, to infuse at 700 U/hr, and nitroglycerin.

1. Identify the nursing assessments that you will perform.

2. Identify the complications that can result from thrombophlebitis.

3. Explain the physiologic bases for each of the following treatment measures:

   a. deep breathing

   b. Kendal alternating pressure stockings

   c. heparin/nitrogylcerin

   d. bed rest

4. What would help prevent a recurrence of the thrombophlebitis?

5. Identify how rapidly the IV should be run to administer the correct amount of heparin (using macrodrop tubing, 10 gtts/mL).

S.K.'s chest pain worsens during the night.

6. Describe what you will do.

S.K. is transferred to ICU with a diagnosis of pulmonary emboli.

7. Can she receive tPA?

S.K. is to go home, and the physician orders Lovenox.

8. What instructions should you give S.K.?

■ Antidysrhythmics: Critical Thinking Case Study

Mr. C. is a 65-year-old man who weighs 150 lb and has a 20-year history of COPD. He is brought to the ER complaining of chest pain and severe shortness of breath. He is diagnosed with pneumonia and heart failure.

1. Identify what your initial assessments and nursing actions will be for this client.

2. The dysrhythmia above is _____.

3. Identify how and why this dysrhythmia must be treated.

6. Describe the side effects that you will be assessing for.

The doctor chooses to treat the dysrhythmia with digoxin.

4. Describe the digitalizing routine.

Despite treatment, Mr. C. is still experiencing the same dysrhythmia.

7. Discuss other alternative treatments.

While in the ER, Mr. C's rhythm changes.

5. Identify the medication that you would administer and how it is to be administered.

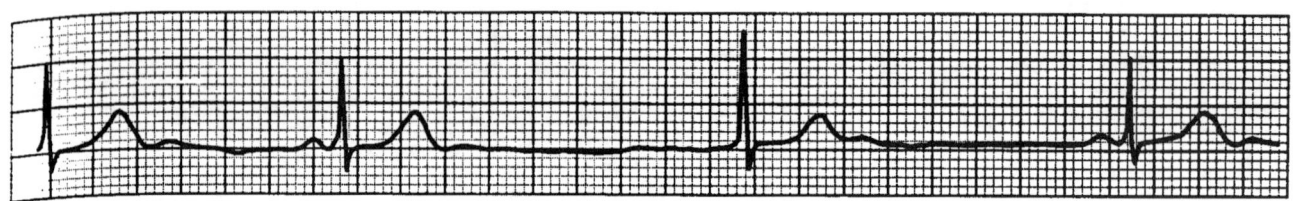

Finally, Mr. C. converts to sinus rhythms, but his rate is low.

8. Identify the dysrhythmia above. _____

9. Identify your nursing responsibilities.

Electrolytes are drawn, and the results are K^+ 5.3, Na^+ 130, and creatinine 2.6

10. Identify what you should be assessing for.

The physician orders Dobutamine, 250 mg in 250 mL D5W, to run at 10 μg/kg/min, Lasix 80 mg IV push, KCl 40 mEq (10 mEq in 50 mL each hour for next 4 hours), and morphine 2 mg IV push.

11. Identify why these medications were ordered and why they are being administered in such a manner.

12. Identify the volume per hour at which you will set the infusion pump to deliver the correct amount of dobutamine.

After Lasix is administered, Mr. C.'s BP drops to 80/50. An IV drip of dopamine is started to maintain his blood pressure at 100/60.

13. Identify why it is important to maintain Mr. C.'s BP above 100.

Drug Calculations

1. Order: Give 1300 mg of calcium carbonate.
   Available: 648 mg/tablet.
   Administer: _____ tablets.

2. Order: Give 250 mg of Diocto-Liquid.
   Available: 50 mg/5 mL.
   Administer: _____ mL.

3. Order: Give 2 tsp of Phanatuss cough syrup.
   Administer: _____ mL.

4. Order: Give 0.3 mL of SSKI.
   Available: 1 g/mL.
   Administer: _____ mg.

5. Order: Give 400 mg of Tagamet.
   Available: 300 mg/5 mL
   Administer: _____ mL.

6. Order: Give 650 mg of acetaminophen.
   Available: 160 mg/5 mL.
   Administer: _____ mL.

7. Order: 1000 mL D5W to run for 12 hours.
   Available: Tubing that delivers 10 drops = 1 mL.
   Delivery rate: _____ mL/hr.
   Delivery rate: _____ drops/min.

8. Order: 3 liters of IV solution to run for 24 hours.
   Available: Tubing that delivers 15 drops = 1 mL.
   Delivery rate: _____ mL/hr.
   Delivery rate: _____ drops/min.

9. Order: 250 mL of D5W at 30 mL/hr.
   Available: Tubing that delivers 60 drops = 1 mL.
   Delivery rate: _____ drops/min.

10. Order: 1000 mL of D5W with 10 mEq KCl over
    10 hours.
    Available: KCl 60 mEq/30 mL vial; tubing that
    delivers 15 drops = 1 mL.
    Inject into IV bag: _____ mL.
    Delivery rate: _____ drops/min.

11. A liter of IV fluid is started at 9 AM and is to run
    for 8 hours. The IV is discontinued at 1 PM.
    How much fluid is left? _____ mL.

12. Order: IV (piggyback) of gentamicin in 50 mL
    D5W over 20 minutes.
    Available: Macrodrop set (10 drops = 1 mL).
    Delivery rate: _____ drops/min.

13. Order: Heparin sodium 3000 U SC.
    Available: Heparin sodium 10,000 U/mL.
    Administer: _____ mL.

14. Order: Demerol 75 mg, Atropine 0.25 mg IM,
    Vistaril 12.5 mg.
    Available: Demerol 50 mg/mL, Atropine 0.4
    mg/mL, Vistaril 25 mg/mL.
    Administer: _____ mL Demerol.
    Administer: _____ mL Atropine.
    Administer: _____ mL Vistaril.
    Can these medications be administered in the
    same syringe? _____.

15. Order: Phenytoin 75 mg IV.
    Available: Phenytoin (Dilantin) 250 mg/5 mL.
    Administer: _____ mL.

16. Order: Aminophylline 300 mg PO.
    Available: 500 mg/20 mL.
    Administer: _____ mL.

17. Order: Heparin 20,000 U in 1000 mL D5W at 50
    mL/hr.
    Delivery rate: _____ U/hr.

18. Order: Nitroprusside 100 mg in 250 mL D5W at 50 mL/hr.
    Delivery rate: _____ mg/hr.

19. Order: Nitroprusside 50 mg in 250 mL D5W at 100 mcg/min.
    Delivery rate: _____ mL/hr.

20. Order: Dopamine 400 mg in 250 mL D5W at 320 mcg/min.
    Delivery rate: _____ mL/hr.

21. Order: Norepinephrine 2 mg in 250 mL D5W at 25 mL/hr.
    Delivery rate: _____ mcg/hr.

22. Order: Dobutamine 1000 mg in 500 mL D5W at 20 mL/hr.
    Delivery rate: _____ mg/hr.

23. Order: Dobutamine 250 mg in 250 mL of D5W at 20 mL/hr.
    Delivery rate: _____ mg/min.

24. Order: Lidocaine 1 g in 250 mL D5W at 2 mg/min.
    Available: Microdrip tubing (60 drops = 1 mL).
    Delivery rate: _____ drops/min.

25. Order: Dopamine 400 mg in 500 mL D5W at 60 mL/hr.
    Delivery rate: _____ mg/hr.

26. Order: Isoproterenol 5 mg in 500 mL D5W at 50 mL/hr.
    Delivery rate: _____ mg/hr.

27. Order: Aminophylline 250 mg in 500 mL D5W at 25 mL/hr.
    Delivery rate: _____ mg/hr.

28. Order: Regular insulin 100 U in 250 mL D5W at 30 mL/hr.

    Delivery rate: _____ U/hr.

29. Order: Lidocaine 1 g in 1000 mL D5W at 60 mL/hr.

    Delivery rate: _____ mg/min.

30. Order: Streptokinase 750,000 U in 50 mL over 30 minutes.

    Delivery rate: _____ U/min.

Answers

Chapter 1

MATCHING EXERCISE (TERMS AND CONCEPTS)
1. D.	2. E.	3. A.	4. G.	5. B.
6. K.	7. I.	8. F.	9. H.	10. C.
11. J.	12. O.	13. L.	14. M.	15. N.

FILL IN THE BLANKS

CELL PHYSIOLOGY, PART I

1. Cell membrane
2. Cytoplasm
3. Lysosomes
4. Nucleus
5. Chromatin
6. Endoplasmic reticulum
7. Ribosomes
8. Golgi apparatus
9. Mitochondria

CELL PHYSIOLOGY, PART II

1. Drug movement and therefore drug action are affected by a drug's ability to cross cell membranes.
2. Prostaglandins and histamine are released in response to cellular damage and cause vasodilation, vascular permeability, pain and edema.

SOURCE OF DRUGS
1. a. plants
   b. animals
   c. minerals
2. a. synthetic chemical compounds derived from technology

REVIEW QUESTIONS
1. a.	2. a.	3. a.	4. c.	5. c.
6. a.	7. a.	8. d.	9. b.	10. b.

Chapter 2

FILL IN THE BLANKS
1. cross cell membranes.
2. Lipid, water.
3. Dosage.
4. slows.
5. lungs, mucous membranes.
6. adequacy of circulation.
7. protein binding.
8. unbound.
9. blood-brain barrier.
10. Metabolism.
11. enzymes, liver.
12. enzyme induction.
13. kidneys, bowel, lungs, skin.
14. enzymes, proteins.
15. stimulate, inhibit.
16. number of receptor sites.
17. chemical structure.
18. administration, absorption, distribution.
19. neonates, infants, liver, kidney.
20. activation of drug metabolizing enzymes which accelerate drug metabolism and excretion.

DEFINITIONS
1. Movement of a drug from an area of higher concentration to an area of lower concentration.
2. Drug molecules move from an area of lower concentration to an area of higher concentration.
3. The elimination of a drug from the body.
4. The time required for the serum concentration of a drug to be decreased by 50%.
5. Drugs that produce effects similar to those produced by naturally occurring hormones, neurotransmitters, and other substances.
6. Drugs that inhibit cell function by occupying receptor sites.
7. Results when two drugs are taken together, producing a greater effect than when either drug is taken alone.
8. An unexpected reaction to a drug taken for the first time.
9. Drugs stimulate liver cells to produce larger amounts of drug metabolizing enzymes.
10. Fever associated with the administration of medication.

MATCHING EXERCISE (TERMS AND CONCEPTS)
1. B.	2. C.	3. D.	4. A.

REVIEW QUESTIONS
1. b.	2. d.	3. b.	4. b.	5. c.
6. c.	7. b.	8. d.	9. b.	10. a.

Chapter 3

MATCHING EXERCISE (TERMS AND CONCEPTS)
1. B.	2. F.	3. A.	4. C.	5. D.
6. E.	7. G.	8. H.	9. I.	10. J.
11. L.	12. O.	13. M.	14. N.	15. P.
16. R.	17. K.	18. S.	19. U.	20. V.

ABBREVIATIONS

1. I.	2. F.	3. G.	4. C.	5. J.
6. E.	7. B.	8. D.	9. H.	10. A.

EQUIVALENTS

1. E.	2. C.	3. H.	4. K.	5. A.
6. D.	7. B.	8. F.	9. G.	10. L.

DIAGRAM

Subcutaneous injections

PRACTICE QUESTIONS (MEDICATION ORDERS)

1. b.	2. a.	3. c.

DOSAGE CALCULATIONS (PRACTICE SET I)

1. 2 tablets.
2. 0.25 mL.
3. 60 mL.
4. 3 tablets.
5. 0.5 cc.
6. 0.4 cc.
7. 1.25 mL.
8. 8 cc.
9. 4 mL.
10. 0.5 cc.

DOSAGE CALCULATIONS (PRACTICE SET II)

1. 60 mL.
2. 3 tablets.
3. 360 mL.
4. 60 kg.
5. 1250 mL.
6. 2.5 mL.
7. 1.2 g.
8. 0.4 mL.
9. 0.25 mL.
10. 2 tsp.

REVIEW QUESTIONS (DOSAGE CALCULATIONS)

1. a.	2. a.	3. d.	4. b.	5. c.
6. a.	7. a.	8. b.	9. b.	10. b.

Chapter 4

TRUE OR FALSE

1. T.	2. F.	3. T.	4. T.	5. T.
6. F.	7. T.	8. T.	9. F.	10. T.
11. T.	12. F.	13. T.	14. T.	15. T.

REVIEW QUESTIONS

1. c.	2. d.	3. b.	4. c.	5. d.
6. a.	7. b.	8. b.	9. d.	10. b.

Chapter 5

FILL IN THE BLANKS

1. brain, spinal cord.
2. ability to produce an action potential.
3. ability to convey electrical impulses.
4. amines, amino acids, peptides.
5. dopamine, norepinephrine, serotonin
6. conscious processes.
7. heat, cold, pain, position sense.
8. water balance, body temperature, hormone levels, arterial blood pressure, heart rate, other body functions
9. cardiac, respiratory, vasomotor.
10. wakefulness, alertness.
11. feeding behavior, wake sleep cycles, emotions, behavior.
12. muscular activity, balance, posture.
13. skeletal muscle.
14. medulla.
15. hypoxia.
16. confusion, dizziness, convulsions, loss of consciousness, brain damage.
17. Thiamine.
18. myelin sheaths, Wernicke-Korsakoff.
19. drowsiness, decreased muscle tone, decreased ability to move, decreased perception of sensation.
20. unconsciousness, respiratory failure, death.
21. wakefulness, alertness, decreased fatigue.
22. hyperactivity, excessive talking, nervousness, insomnia.
23. seizures, dysrhythmias, death.

NEUROTRANSMISSION, PART I

1. Synapse.
2. Release site.
3. Postsynaptic nerve terminal.
4. Receptor sites.
5. Postsynaptic nerve cell membrane.
6. Presynaptic nerve cell membrane.
7. Neurotransmitters.
8. Presynaptic nerve terminal.

NEUROTRANSMISSION, PART II

1. synapse, receptors.
2. receptor sites.

REVIEW QUESTIONS

1. c.	2. b.	3. d.	4. d.	5. a.
6. d.	7. a.	8. c.	9. a.	10. d.

Chapter 6

FILL IN THE BLANKS

1. a. Drowsiness and unconsciousness.
   b. Decreased mental and physical activity.
   c. Respiratory depression.
   d. Nausea and vomiting.
   e. Pupil constriction.
2. slowing motility, constipation.
3. PO, IM, IV, SC, Epidural, Intrathecal, Rectal.
4. 20 mg, 30 mg.
5. Transmucosal formulation, transdermal patch, 3 days.
6. Tylenol.
7. short acting, less smooth muscle spasm, 50–100 mg, 2–4.
8. Stadol, Nubain, Talwin.
9. Narcan, Revex, Revia.
10. assess the patient's pain.
11. location, intensity or severity, relation to time and activity, other symptoms.
12. ambulation, heat or cold, relaxation.
13. IV, it is faster acting.
14. PCA pump.
15. suppository, patches.
16. Atropine.
17. crying, thrashing, muscle rigidity.
18. Opioid rectal.
19. sedation, confusion, urinary retention.
20. hepatic.
21. drowsiness, weakness, unsteady gait, blurred vision.

WORD FIND

1. Fentanyl.
2. Codeine.
3. Demerol.
4. Dilaudid.
5. Morphine.
6. Stadol.
7. Darvon.
8. Nubain.
9. Narcan.
10. Talwin.

REVIEW QUESTIONS

1. d.	2. a.	3. b.	4. a.	5. d.
6. a.	7. b.	8. d.	9. d.	10. c.

Chapter 7

MATCHING EXERCISE (TERMS AND CONCEPTS)

1. D.	2. E.	3. A.	4. I.	5. H.
6. B.	7. G.	8. C.	9. F.	10. K.

TRUE OR FALSE

1. T.	2. F.	3. F.	4. T.	5. T.
6. T.	7. T.	8. F.	9. T	10. T
11. T.	12. T.			

REVIEW QUESTIONS

1. d.	2. a.	3. d.	4. c.	5. b.
6. a.	7. a.	8. b.	9. b.	10. c.

CHAPTER 6 WORD FIND

```
N O T H S B H Y P O F T I L C L C E F G H H J N K
K A D R E N E R G I C E N B E T A Z O L O L A N E
C M R I A S S A N L L X Q K E Z S V C D N C A T V
X Y Z T I P L D N E D R O N O N I R L A R N V R R
H L P O D I L A U D I D I C A Y Y O D A V V P P J
F N V A N L I C B R E E K X F H T G N A E S O S B
R I L U A A C A I D D U K L O E E U E T O R R P
X T O S H R F R N O H A Z Y P X D K B B L K A O T
L R N A Y J R E C L N O S T Y H P E A N B E R E C
V A S G O N I Q P F E N T A N Y L K I S N L O K C
X T K X T G A A N G N P A P E C O R N I U O U S A
K J K X C Z A B T N T A D P V C D T E G F G X H O
V A S D I P I O C P R A O Z O I N J K A J K L D N
O N A E S O R P T I O N L W N C I N U C N C I V O
P T O M I I A N G I N Y B W I X K U N L S I N E T
A Z A E Y B I D L E S X F N I N S V D F H I A N I
R S C R F X Z Y N G R H V T G N J N A A E Z H T L
G E M O R P H I N E V K O N M H C H L O R Z I D E
Y N O L G D B P Q E R R O T V S P Q Y L O V B P C
L W I E F I C D L S N E V H O W G Y O Z A J O W D
F D O M R G G L I I S T P R O T E R E N E R Z N X
N C O E U M A D I N S F T P T M I G J F U W T C Y
E F D D Q C N Q N T A T D Y M N S J Z E B G O G C
```

Chapter 8

FILL IN THE BLANKS

1. severe or prolonged.
2. phobias, panic, obsessive-compulsive, posttraumatic stress syndrome, atypical anxiety disorders, general anxiety.
3. (Rapid eye movement), mentally and emotionally restorative.
4. pain, anxiety, illness, changes in lifestyle, drugs.
5. Benzodiazepines, barbiturates.
6. suppression of REM sleep, enzyme induction, tolerance, dependence.
7. physical, psychological.
8. fat, plasma proteins.
9. long, 5–7.
10. (BuSpar), sedation, physical, psychological, muscle relaxant, anticonvulsant.
11. (Vistaril), antiemetic, antihistamine.
12. Chloral hydrate, safe, inexpensive, tolerance.
13. Diphenhydramine (Benadryl).
14. antianxiety, hypnotic, anticonvulsant, agitation, delirium tremens.
15. severe respiratory disorders, severe liver disease, severe kidney disease, hypersensitivity reactions, drug abuse.
16. increased anxiety, insomnia, irritability, headaches, tremor, palpitations, agitation, confusion, abnormal perception of movement, depersonalization, psychosis, seizures.
17. Flumazenil (Romazicon).
18. oxazepam (Serax), lorazepam (Ativan).

DEFINITIONS

1. A response to a stressful situation resulting in fear, apprehension, nervousness, or worry.
2. Prolonged difficulty sleeping or staying asleep.
3. A period of 5–20 minutes of rapid eye movement, dreaming and increased physiologic activity.
4. Stimulation of liver cells to produce large amounts of drug metabolizing enzymes.

NURSING DIAGNOSIS (NURSING DIAGNOSIS)

1. Sleep pattern disturbance, insomnia.
2. Ineffective individual coping.
3. Knowledge deficit related to the appropriate use of antianxiety medication.

NURSING DIAGNOSIS (ASSESSMENT DATA)

1. Observe for physiological manifestations of anxiety: increased BP, pulse, respirations, and muscle tension.
2. a. Assess level of anxiety.
   b. Assess effects of anxiety on perception, ability to learn, and problem solving.
3. Assess for a therapeutic response to the medication.

NURSING DIAGNOSIS (NURSING INTERVENTIONS)

1. a. Reduce environmental stimuli.
   b. Use measures to increase comfort.
   c. Administer antianxiety medication.
2. a. Remain calm.
   b. Assist client to identify stressors.
   c. Provide outlets for excess energy.
   d. Identify previous coping mechanisms.
3. a. Instruct client to avoid alcohol while using the medication.
   b. Instruct client that antianxiety medications are for short-term use.
   c. Assess client knowledge regarding the medications.

REVIEW QUESTIONS

1. d.	2. b.	3. a.	4. c.	5. a.
6. b.	7. a.	8. c.	9. c.	10. c.

Chapter 9

FILL IN THE BLANKS

1. Psychosis.
2. Hallucinations.
3. Delusions.
4. schizophrenia.
5. Schizophrenia.
6. physical disorders, drug intoxication and drug withdrawal.
7. CNS depression, autonomic nervous system depression, antiemetic effect, lowering of body temperature, hypersensitivity reactions.
8. dopamine.
9. anxiety, agitation, hyperactivity, insomnia, hallucinations, aggressive/combative.
10. nausea, vomiting.
11. (Phenergan), sedative, antiemetic, antihistaminic.
12. (Taractan), (Navane), antipsychotic.
13. (Haldol), low, hypotension, sedation, high, extrapyramidal effects.
14. mental retardation with hyperkinesia, Tourette's syndrome, Huntington's disease.
15. acute dystonia, parkinsonism, akathisia, tardive dyskinesia.
16. (Loxitane), (Clozaril), agranulocytosis, constipation, dizziness, hypotension, seizures.
17. Tourette's syndrome, tardive dyskinesia, major motor seizures, sudden death.
18. alleviate symptoms, increase the client's ability to cope, promote optimal functioning.
19. another psychiatric drug, reappearance of symptoms.
20. injections, fluphenazine (Prolixin).
21. once, bedtime.
22. more rapidly, adverse reactions.
23. slowly, higher.
24. confusion, memory impairment, hallucinations, constipation, urinary retention, and heat stroke.
25. dental check-ups, tooth brushing, drinking fluids, rinsing mouth.

CAUTION OR CONTRAINDICATION

1. ci.	2. ci.	3. ci.	4. ca.	5. ca.
6. ci.	7. ca.	8. ca.	9. ci.	10. ci.
11. ca.	12. ci.	13. ci.		

CHAPTER 9 WORD FIND

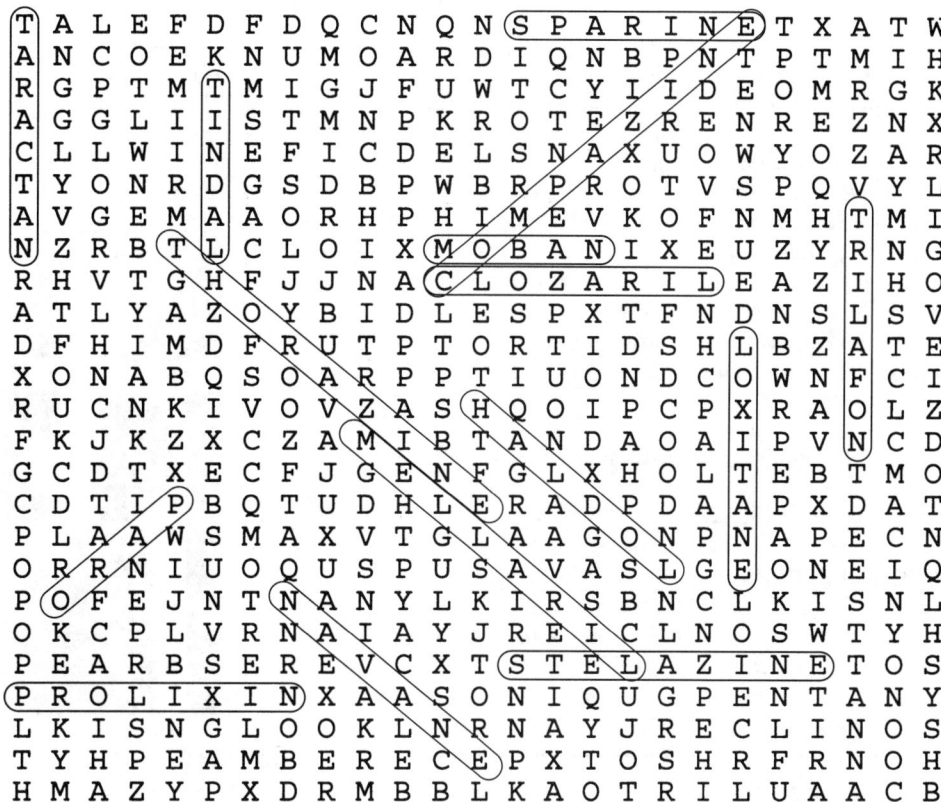

WORD FIND

1. Tindal.
2. Mellaril.
3. Compazine.
4. Prolixin.
5. Thorazine.
6. Trilafon.
7. Sparine.
8. Stelazine.
9. Moban.
10. Orap.
11. Clozaril.
12. Haldol.
13. Taractan.
14. Navane.
15. Loxitane.

REVIEW QUESTIONS

1. d.   2. d.   3. c.   4. b.   5. b.
6. a.   7. b.   8. c.   9. d.   10. d.

Chapter 10

FILL IN THE BLANKS

1. a. Fatigue.
   b. Indecisiveness.
   c. Difficulty concentrating.
   d. Loss of interest in appearance.
   e. Loss of interest in work.
   f. Loss of interest in sex.
   g. Feelings of guilt.

   h. Change in appetite.
   i. Sleep disorder.
   j. Somatic symptoms.
   k. Obsession with death.
2. environmental stress, adverse life events, drugs, concurrent disease states.
3. sedation, orthostatic hypotension.
4. (Elavil), TCA.
5. (Prozac), nausea, nervousness, insomnia, skin rash.
6. 2–3 months.
7. foods, drugs, hypertensive crisis.
8. tyramine.
9. a. Cheese.
   b. Alcohol.
   c. Bananas.
   d. Caffeine.
   e. Chocolate.
   f. Raisins.
   g. Sour cream.
   h. Yogurt.
10. (Eskalith), bipolar affective disorder.
11. Adequate kidney function.
12. sodium.
13. 5–7.
14 bed wetting.
15. a lifetime.
16. 2–3.
17. nausea, vomiting, agitation, restlessness, hypomania.
18. nystagmus, tremors, oliguria, confusion, impaired consciousness, hallucinations, choreiform movements, convulsions, coma, death.

SENTENCE CORRECTION

1. Urinary retention; *circle* insomnia.
2. Meperidine (Demerol); *circle* Furosemide (Lasix). Or: Adrenergic agents, alcohol, guanethidine, levodopa, and reserpine.
3. Sodium; *circle* potassium.
4. Daily; *circle* b.i.d.
5. Severe headaches; *circle* Blurred vision.
6. Renal; *circle* hepatic.
7. Norepinephrine and serotonin; *circle* dopamine.
8. Arrhythmias; *circle* failure.
9. Hemodialysis; *circle* Gastric lavage.
10. SSRIs; *circle* TCAs.
11. 4; *circle* 8.
12. Mania; *circle* depression.
13. hypotension; *circle* hypertension.
14. 2; *circle* 6.
15. 12, 6; *circle* 18, 12.

REVIEW QUESTIONS

1. d.   2. d.   3. a.   4. d.   5. d.
6. d.   7. b.   8. d.   9. b.   10. c.

Chapter 11

FILL IN THE BLANKS

1. brief episode of abnormal electrical activity.
2. type of seizure characterized by spasmodic contractions of involuntary muscles.
3. chronic, recurrent pattern of seizures.
4. EEG.
5. developmental defects, metabolic disease, birth injury.
6. cocaine, lidocaine, theophylline.
7. ataxia, drowsiness, lethargy, nausea, vomiting, gingival hyperplasia.
8. Carbamazepine, psychomotor, tonic-clonic, mixed, trigeminal neuralgia.
9. (Valium), (Ativan), acute convulsive seizures.
10. brain surgery, head injury, drug overdose.
11. life long.
12. weeks or months.
13. decrease effects of dopamine; bradycardia, heart block.
14. lorazepam (Ativan).
15. folic acid.

TRUE OR FALSE

1. T.   2. F.   3. F.   4. T.   5. F.
6. F.   7. T.

CROSSWORD PUZZLE

ACROSS

2. Klonopin.
4. Tranxene.
5. Valium.
9. Phenobarbital.

DOWN

1. Convulsion.
3. Tegretol.
6. Dilantin.
7. Depakene.
8. Epilepsy.
10. Ativan.

REVIEW QUESTIONS

1. a.   2. a.   3. b.   4. b.   5. c.
6. a.   7. a.   8. d.   9. c.   10. c.

Chapter 12

FILL IN THE BLANKS

1. chronic, progressive, degenerative; tremor, bradykinesia, joint and muscle rigidity.
2. dopamine producing nerve cells.
3. (Dopar, Larodopa), (Lodosyn), (Symmetrel), (Parlodel), (Permax), (Mirapex), (Requip), (Eldepryl), and (Tasmar).
4. (Symmetrel), dopamine release.
5. postsynaptic dopamine receptors.
6. MAO B, inactivates.
7. COMT
8. most effective.
9. recurrence.
10. Sinemet, brain.
11. (Symmetrel), 1–5.
12. dopamine receptors.
13. (Mirapex), (Requip), beginning, advanced.

TRUE OR FALSE

1. F.   2. T.   3. T.   4. F.   5. T.
6. F.   7. T.

REVIEW QUESTIONS

1. d.   2. d.   3. b.   4. c.   5. a.
6. c.   7. d.   8. b.   9. b.   10. c.

Chapter 13

FILL IN THE BLANKS
1 decrease muscle spasms, spasticity.
2. Dantrolene (Dantrium).
3. hyperthermia.
4. Diazepam (Valium), methocarbamol (Robaxin).
5. baclofen (Lioresal).
6. a. Massage, moist heat, and exercise.
   b. Bed rest for acute muscle spasm.
   c. Relaxation techniques.
   d. Correct posture and lifting.
7. Children.
8. mental alertness, physical coordination.
9. food or milk, nausea.
10. (Lioresal), hallucinations.

TRUE OR FALSE
1. T.   2. F.   3. F.   4. T.   5. F.   6. F.

CROSSWORD PUZZLE

ACROSS
2. Dizziness.
3. Baclofen.
4. Chlorphenesin.
6. Spasticity.
8. Dantrolene.
9. Pregnancy.
10. Methocarbamol.

DOWN
1. Massage.
5. Orphenadrine.
7. Diazepam.

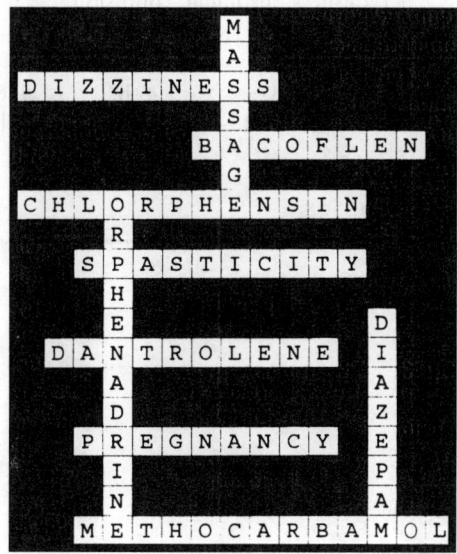

REVIEW QUESTIONS
1. b.   2. d.   3. d.   4. a.   5. b.
6. d.   7. d.   8. a.   9. d.   10. d.

Chapter 14

MATCHING EXERCISE (TERMS AND CONCEPTS)
1. B.	2. A.	3. E.	4. C.	5. I.
6. K.	7. H.	8. G.	9. D.	10. F.
11. L.	12. M.	13. N.	14. O.	15. P.

WORD SCRAMBLE
1. Ethrane.
2. Forane.
3. Alfenta.
4. Innovar.
5. Pavulon.
6. Anectine.
7. Metubine.
8. Sufenta.
9. Versed.
10. Brevital.

REVIEW QUESTIONS
1. b.	2. d.	3. d.	4. a.	5. a.
6. c.	7. c.	8. d.	9. a.	10. a.

Chapter 15

MATCHING EXERCISE (TERMS AND CONCEPTS)
1. B.	2. C.	3. E.	4. G.	5. A.
6. F.	7. I.	8. D.	9. H.	10. J.
11. K.	12. M.	13. L.	14. O.	15. N.
16. P				

NURSING DIAGNOSIS (NURSING DIAGNOSIS)
1. Alteration in nutrition: malnutrition and vitamin deficiencies.
2. Risk for violence related to altered thought process.
3. Decreased cardiac output associated with fluid volume excess.
4. Risk for injury related to bleeding.

NURSING DIAGNOSIS (ASSESSMENT DATA)
1. Lab studies to assess for anemia and electrolyte imbalances. Assess client for signs/symptoms of a deficiency.
2. Assess client for impaired motor coordination, poor task performance, and hypo/hyperactivity.
3. Assess heart sounds, lung sounds, and ECG. Assess lab studies and serum albumin levels.
4. Assess platelet count and clotting studies.

NURSING DIAGNOSIS (NURSING INTERVENTIONS)
1. Administer folic acid, thiamine, and vitamin B_{12}.
2. Administer sedative. Decrease environmental stimuli. Teach nondrug coping techniques.
3. q4h vs, peripheral pulses. Administer diuretics if appropriate. I & O, daily weights.
4. Observe client for bruising.

CHAPTER 14 WORD FIND

```
B A E C C T R I S O M E T A L C H E M P N I P A N
A L T B A C I T R E M E N A R C H O R O L A C O L
C M H T R A L C O H V P E R A G A R I R I H O K C
F O R A N E R L L S S N E S S T I T H E O P H Y L
T S A N S E I O E A A A N I N N O V A R E A N I X
O C N E T I P N E L A T I E N T G E O M T R I C U
B A E A L N P A L P I T F T I O N S E C O E S N E
A N E B O N D I H E X L L G H A L A B F I N I A X
C N U C T E C H Y P A V U L O N V E R E F L E X E
K A P T A B R A P P R E M E N E I O N T A O V A N
H A H S O M T R E M O R A N G C N E J T A O C N I
A B O T P E P I R N N Q B B A T R I P C O C T N
N C R V Q T I H T E A B I E F I A R E S T L Y H H
E N I M O R B O E H T C N X O N T S E N I M A I C
C I A N S A N T N T A I N T M E T U B I N E M N Y
T A Y N A Z I T S L A E M O R D N F S S E T T E R
O M A H V O T R A C O M M R E X N E O E I F I N T
P P T A M L R T O P A M I N E C T N L B G N O I S
A H A A D O I C N A A F N N F D D T O E V E S O I
N A T I N V E R S E D I F A E L A A M M P A L O C
T I R E E S T L E S S N E S S U A A W I T O O M C
R R F R C S E T R E O N P I I A U N U T W R I M C
Y B B L R S H N V R R S I S E N I K R E P Y H C A
X T E L B E J Q U T H Y P O A C E B R S H I S P W
A L B E L L A D O W D Y M N T E S O O T Y P A K T
```

DEFINITIONS

1. A chronic, progressive, potentially fatal disease characterized by physical dependence and physiologic changes related to the ingestion of alcohol.
2. Feelings of satisfaction and pleasure from taking a drug.
3. Physiologic adaptation to chronic drug use resulting in uncomfortable symptoms when the drug is stopped.

9. (Dopram), 5–10.
10. analgesia, migraine headaches.
11. neonates.
12. tolerance, psychological dependence, habituation.
13. caffeine.
14. grows, hepatic metabolism.
15. anxiety, nervousness, insomnia, confusion.

REVIEW QUESTIONS

1. a.	2. a.	3. c.	4. c.	5. b.
6. c.	7. b.	8. d.	9. c.	10. a.

REVIEW QUESTIONS

1. b.	2. c.	3. a.	4. b.	5. c.
6. d.	7. a.	8. d.	9. c.	10. b.

Chapter 16

FILL IN THE BLANKS

1. narcolepsy, ADHD (attention deficit-hyperactivity disorder).
2. a rare disorder characterized.
3. children, hyperactivity, a short attention span, difficulty completing assigned tasks, restlessness, impulsive behavior.
4. mood elevation, increased mental alertness, increased capacity for work, heart rate, blood pressure, mydriasis, gastrointestinal motility, behavioral symptoms, increase performance.
5. respiration, seizures.
6. mental alertness, drowsiness.
7. cardiac output, heart rate, diuresis, pepsin, hydrochloric acid.
8. (Ritalin), 5–10 mg, 60 mg.

Chapter 17

FILL IN THE BLANKS

1. Constricts.
2. Decreases.
3. Decreases.
4. Constricts.
5. Increases.
6. Constricts.
7. No effect.
8. Dilates.
9. Increases.
10. Increases.
11. Dilates.
12. Increases.
13. Dilates.
14. Increases.

TRUE OR FALSE

| 1. T. | 2. T. | 3. F. | 4. F. | 5. F. |
| 6. F. | 7. T. | 8. T. | | |

REVIEW QUESTIONS

| 1. c. | 2. d. | 3. c. | 4. a. | 5. b. |
| 6. b. | 7. a. | 8. c. | 9. c. | 10. d. |

Chapter 18

MATCHING EXERCISE (TERMS AND CONCEPTS)

| 1. C. | 2. D. | 3. A. | 4. F. | 5. E. |
| 6. B. | 7. I. | 8. G. | 9. H. | 10. J. |

TRUE OR FALSE

| 1. T. | 2. F. | 3. F. | 4. T. | 5. T. |
| 6. T. | 7. F. | 8. F. | 9. T. | 10. T. |

SENTENCE CORRECTION

1. Isoproterenol (Isuprel); *circle* Ephedrine.
2. Anaphylactic; *circle* allergic.
3. Allergens; *circle* toxins.
4. Acidosis; *circle* Alkalosis.
5. 30; *circle* 5.
6. Epinephrine; *circle* Levarterenol (Levophed).
7. Stimulants; *circle* depressants.
8. Phenylephrine; *circle* Ephedrine.
9. Tachycardia; *circle* bradycardia.
10. Terbutaline (Brethine); *circle* Isoproternol (Isuprel).
11. Blood pressure; *circle* breathing.
12. Rebound nasal congestion; *circle* hypotension.
13. Urinary output; *circle* respiratory status.
14. Increase; *circle* decrease.
15. Hypotension and shock; *circle* bronchodilation and vasoconstriction.

REVIEW QUESTIONS

| 1. b. | 2. a. | 3. a. | 4. b. | 5. c. |
| 6. c. | 7. a. | 8 a. | 9. a. | 10. d. |

Chapter 19

MATCHING EXERCISE (TERMS AND CONCEPTS)

| 1. E. | 2. F. | 3. A. | 4. D. | 5. B. |
| 6. C. | 7. I. | 8. G. | 9. H. | 10. J. |

TRUE OR FALSE

| 1. F. | 2. F. | 3. T. | 4. T. | 5. T. |
| 6. T. | 7. T. | 8. T. | 9. T. | 10. F. |

FILL IN THE BLANKS

1. Epinephrine and norepinephrine.
2. Beta-adrenergic blocking drug.
3. Nerve endings.
4. Receptor site on cell surface.
5. Myocardial or other tissue cells.

SENTENCE CORRECTION

1. Propranolol (Inderal); *circle* Nadolol (Corgard).
2. Selective; *circle* nonselective.
3. Supraventricular tachycardia; *circle* hypertension.
4. Timolol (Timoptic); *circle* pindolol (Visken).
5. Propranolol (Inderal); *circle* levobunolol (Betagan).
6. Tamsulosin (Flomax); *circle* Metoprolol (Lopressor).
7. Atenolol (Tenormin); *circle* penbutolol (Levatol).
8. Nonselective; *circle* Selective.
9. Propranolol (Inderal); *circle* levobunolol (Betagan).
10. myocardial infarction; *circle* stroke.
11. Decreasing; *circle* increasing.
12. Beta$_1$; *circle* beta$_2$.
13. Bradycardia; *circle* tachycardia.
14. Lipid; *circle* water.
15. Decreased; *circle* increased.

REVIEW QUESTIONS

| 1. a. | 2. c. | 3. a. | 4. c. | 5. d. |
| 6. a. | 7. d. | 8. c. | 9. a. | 10. d. |

Chapter 20

FILL IN THE BLANKS

1. a. decreased.
   b. increased.
   c. relaxation of.
   d. increased.
   e. increased.
   f. increased.
   g. constriction of.

MATCHING EXERCISE (TERMS AND CONCEPTS)

| 1. D. | 2. A. | 3. B. | 4. C. | 5. E. |

TRUE OR FALSE

| 1. T. | 2. T. | 3. F. | 4. T. | 5. T. |

REVIEW QUESTIONS

| 1. a. | 2. c. | 3. a. | 4. b. | 5. c. |
| 6. a. | 7. d. | 8. d. | 9. d. | 10. d. |

Chapter 21

FILL IN THE BLANKS

1. acetylcholine, parasympathetic.
2. a. CNS stimulation followed by CNS depression.
   b. slowed heart rate.
   c. bronchodilation and decreased respiratory tract secretion.
   d. antispasmodic effect in GI tract.
   e. mydriasis and cycloplegia.
   f. decreased secretion of sweat glands.
   g. relaxation of ureters and bladder.
   h. relaxation of smooth muscle of gall bladder and bile ducts.
3. peptic ulcer disease, gastritis, pylorospasm, diverticulitis, ileitis, ulcerative colitis.
4. examination, surgery, mydriatic, cycloplegic.
5. increase.

6. inhalation.
7. salivation, spasticity, tremors.
8. respiratory secretions, vagal stimulation.
9. prostatic hypertrophy, myasthenia gravis, hyperthyroidism, glaucoma, tachyarrhythmias, myocardial infarction, CHF.
10. prototype, PO, IM, IV, SC, topically, inhalation.
11. spasm, increased secretion, increased motility.
12. motion sickness, skin patch, 72.
13. Trihexyphenidyl, parkinsonism, extrapyramidal reactions.
14. Benztropine, acute dystonic reactions.
15. dysuria, urgency, frequency, pain.
16. (Ditropan), bladder capacity, frequency.
17. a. gastrointestinal disorders
    b. genitourinary disorders
    c. ophthalmic disorders
    d. respiratory disorders
    e. bradycardia
    f. Parkinson's disease
18. physostigmine salicylate (Antilirium).
19. facial flushing, skin rash.
20. blurred vision, confusion, heat stroke, constipation, urinary retention, hallucinations, psychotic-like symptoms.

TRUE OR FALSE

| 1. F. | 2. T. | 3. F. | 4. F. | 5. T. |

MATCHING EXERCISE

| 1. C. | 2. D. | 3. A. | 4. B. | 5. E. |
| 6. F. | | | | |

REVIEW QUESTIONS

| 1. c. | 2. d. | 3. c. | 4. c. | 5. d. |
| 6. d. | 7. a. | 8. c. | 9. a. | 10. b. |

Chapter 22

MATCHING EXERCISE (TERMS AND CONCEPTS)

1. D.	2. E.	3. F.	4. I.	5. J.
6. A.	7. B.	8. G.	9. C.	10. H.
11. L.	12. K.	13. M		

TRUE OR FALSE

| 1. T. | 2. F. | 3. T. | 4. F. | 5. T. |
| 6. F. | 7. T. | 8. F. | | |

REVIEW QUESTIONS

| 1. d. | 2. a. | 3. b. | 4. b. | 5. a. |
| 6. d. | 7. b. | 8. b. | 9. a. | 10. a. |

Chapter 23

MATCHING EXERCISE (TERMS AND CONCEPTS)

1. F.	2. A.	3. D.	4. I.	5. H.
6. L.	7. G.	8. B.	9. C.	10. E.
11. J.	12. K.	13. O	14. N.	15. M.

FILL IN THE BLANKS

1. Prolactin.
2. Growth hormone.
3. TSH.
4. ACTH.
5. LH.
6. FSH.
7. ADH.
8. Oxytocin.

REVIEW QUESTIONS

| 1. d. | 2. c. | 3. d. | 4. b. | 5. b. |
| 6. b. | 7. d. | 8. c. | 9. d. | 10. a. |

Chapter 24

TRUE OR FALSE

1. F.	2. F.	3. F.	4. F.	5. T.
6. T.	7. T.	8. T.	9. F.	10. T.
11. T.	12. T.	13. T.	14. T.	15. F.
16. T.	17. T.	18. F.		

CHECKLIST (UNDESIRABLE EFFECTS OF DRUG ADMINISTRATION)

1.	2. ✔	3. ✔	4. ✔	5. ✔
6. ✔	7.	8. ✔	9. ✔	10. ✔
11. ✔	12. ✔	13. ✔	14. ✔	15. ✔
16. ✔	17. ✔	18.	19.	20. ✔
21. ✔	22. ✔	23.	24. ✔	

WORD SCRAMBLE

1. Vanceril.
2. Celestone.
3. Florinef.
4. Aerobid.
5. Aristospan.
6. Cortef.
7. Medrol.
8. Sterane.
9. Cortone.
10. Flonase.
11. Decadron.
12. Aristocort.
13. Hydeltrasol.
14. Deltasone.

REVIEW QUESTIONS

| 1. d. | 2. b. | 3. d. | 4. c. | 5. d. |
| 6. c. | 7. d. | 8. a. | 9. d. | 10. a. |

CHAPTER 24 WORD FIND

```
A P P L H E X N O T H S B H Y P O F T I L C L C E
B F G H D J K A D R E N E R G I C E N B E C T A Z
C O L A E N E C M R A I S S A N L L X Q K O V Z S
D E A N L V C D N C H T N H X Y Z T I P L R D N E
E G G H T D R O E O N I R Y L A R N V R H T L P O
F O N T A D I L N C A Y Y D O D A V P P J O F N V
A N L E S C B R E I K X F E H T G N A E B N O S B
R I F L O R I N E F L U A L A C A A I D A E U K L
O E E U N R E T O R P M X T T O S H R F R N O H A
Y P X C E L E S T O N E D R K B B L K A O T L R N
A J R E C L N O N O T D H A R I S T O C O R T S B
H Y P O F T I L C L C R E S F G H H J N K K A D R
E N E R G I C E L N B O E O T D A Z O L O L A N E
C M R A I S S I A N E L L X E K V Z S X C W C A
H L P O D I R L A U D I D N A C A Y Y O D A U P J
R I L U A E C A A I D A V H A L D R O N X H A P
D K B E C L A O T L R N A Y J D R E C L N O S T Y
M P E N A M B E R E C V A S G R O N I Q P P F E N
T A A E R O B I D N Y L K I G O N L O K C T K X T
G V A A N G A R I S T O S P A N T A P E S C O R N
I U O U S A L E T M O D T I I B T U D H T R P P L
A S O N B S O R P H Y D R O C O C O R T E F I O N
C W A C I N U C N K I X O P T O R I T A R N G I N
Y B P I X K U N L S I N E T A X A A Y B A I D L E
S F N D N S V D F H C I A N I G E M O R N P H A N
K O N M F L O N A S E G D E P E R R T E S P L O
```

Chapter 25

FILL IN THE BLANKS

1. iodine.
2. metabolism, every cell in the body
3. growth, development.
4. poor growth and development, lethargy, inactivity, feeding problems, slow pulse, subnormal temperature, constipation.
5. variable, depending on the amount of thyroid hormone production.
6. nervousness, emotional instability, restlessness, anxiety, insomnia, hyperactive reflexes.
7. tachycardia, fever, dehydration, heart failure, coma.
8. antithyroid drugs, radioactive iodine, surgery, a combination of methods.
9. Levothyroxine (Synthroid), daily, 0.1–0.2 mg.
10. hyperthyroidism.
11. expectorant, in preparation for thyroid surgery.
12. propranolol, (Inderal), tachycardia, palpitations, excessive sweating, tremors, nervousness.
13. .5–5 μg/100 mL.
14. 12.
15. height, weight.
16. 100.

NURSING DIAGNOSIS (NURSING DIAGNOSIS)

1. Altered nutrition: less than body requirement.
2. Altered bowel elimination: diarrhea.
3. Altered comfort related to hypermetabolic state.
4. Knowledge deficit: related to drug therapy.
5. Altered cardiac output.

NURSING DIAGNOSIS (ASSESSMENT DATA)

1. Assess weight.
2. Assess for electrolyte imbalance.
3. Assess nutrition.
4. Assess client's knowledge of medication.
5. Monitor vital signs. Observe for symptoms of CHF.

NURSING DIAGNOSIS (NURSING INTERVENTIONS)

1. Provide extra calories.
2. Instruct to increase fluids. Instruct to avoid foods that cause diarrhea.
3. Instruct to take cool baths and wear lightweight clothing. Instruct to rest.
4. Instruct client regarding antithyroid drugs.
5. Administer propranolol (Inderal) if appropriate.

DEFINITIONS

1. Enlargement of the thyroid gland resulting from iodine deficiency.
2. Occurs as the result of a poorly functioning thyroid gland and results in poor growth and development in children.
3. A condition resulting from hypofunctioning of the thyroid gland.
4. A complication of thyrotoxicosis, symptoms of which include severe tachycardia, fever, dehydration, heart failure, and coma.

REVIEW QUESTIONS

| 1. b. | 2. d. | 3. a. | 4. d. | 5. c. |
| 6. a. | 7. c. | 8. b. | 9. b. | 10. b. |

Chapter 26

FILL IN THE BLANKS

1. parathyroid hormone, calcitonin.
2. up, down.
3. a. increases bone breakdown or reabsorption.
   b. increases absorption of calcium from food.
   c. increases reabsorption of calcium in renal tubules.
4. lowers, bone, serum, long term.
5. foods, exposure to sunlight, serum calcium levels, increasing, mobilizing calcium from bone.
6. calcium, phosphorus.
7. Ricketts.
8. a. cell membrane permeability and function.
   b. nerve cell excitability and transmission of impulses.
   c. contraction of muscles.
   d. blood coagulation and platelet adhesion.
   e. hormone secretion.
   f. enzyme activity.
   g. catecholamine release.
   h. release of chemical mediators.
9. 1000 mg.
10. milk, broccoli, spinach, kale, mustard greens, seafood (clams, oysters).
11. a. is an essential component of DNA, RNA, and other nucleic acids.
    b. combines with fatty acids to form phospholipids, which are required in the structure of all cell membranes.
    c. forms a phosphate buffer system.
    d. is necessary for cell use of glucose.
    e. is necessary for proper function of B vitamins.
12. meat, poultry, fish, eggs, nuts.
13. neuromuscular irritability, tetany.
14. lethargy, confusion.
15. hyperparathyroidism, hyperthyroidism, malignant neoplasms, vitamin D or vitamin A intoxication, aluminum intoxication, prolonged immobilization, adrenocortical insufficiency; thiazide diuretics, estrogen, lithium; cancer.
16. corticosteroids, furosemide (Lasix), phenytoin (Dilantin).
17. lowers.
18. (Lasix), increases.
19. irreversible damage, impairment of functions.
20. blocking resorption from bone.
21. reabsorption of calcium in renal tubules.
22. 3000–4000.

TRUE OR FALSE

1. T.   2. F.   3. T.   4. F.   5. T.

REVIEW QUESTIONS

1 a.   2. a.   3. d.   4. a.   5. b.
6. c.   7. d.   8. c.   9. d.   10. d.

Chapter 27

FILL IN THE BLANKS

1. a. increases.
   b. decreases.
   c. decreases.
   d. increases.
   e. increases.
   f. decreases.
   g. decreases.

MATCHING EXERCISE (TERMS AND CONCEPTS)

1. C.   2. D.   3. F.   4. H.   5. E.
6. I.   7. J.   8. K.   9. M.   10. N.

CROSSWORD PUZZLE

ACROSS

5. Glyburide.
7. Insulin.
8. Glimepiride.
10. Salicylates.
12. Hypoglycemia.

DOWN

1. Human.
2. Ketoacidosis.
3. Rosiglitazone.
4. Acetohexamide.
6. Lipodystrophy.
9. Lipid.

Study Guide to Accompany Clinical Drug Therapy: Rationales for Nursing Practice, sixth edition, by Gail Ropelewski-Ryan.

TRUE OR FALSE

1. T.	2. T.	3. F.	4. T.	5. F.
6. F.	7. T.	8. F.	9. T.	10. T.
11. T.	12. F.	13. T.		

REVIEW QUESTIONS

1. a.	2. d.	3. b.	4. b.	5. d.
6. d.	7. c.	8. c.	9. b.	10. b.

Chapter 28

TRUE OR FALSE

1. T.	2. F.	3. T.	4. T.	5. T.
6. F.	7. T.	8. F.	9. T.	10. F.
11. T.	12. T.	13. T.	14. F.	15. T.

FILL IN THE BLANKS

1. a. atrophic vaginitis
   b. vasomotor instability
   c. osteoporosis
   d. myocardial infarction

NAME THAT DRUG

1. Estradiol transdermal system (Estraderm).
2. Dienestrol (DV).
3. DES (Stilbestrol).
4. Conjugated estrogen (Premarin).
5. Hydroxyprogesterone caproate (Hylutin).
6. Estradiol cypionate (Depo-Estradiol).
7. Norplant.
8. Medroxyprogesterone (Depo-Provera).
9. Megestrol acetate (Megace).
10. Estrogen (Premarin).
11. Oral contraceptives.
12. Estropipate (Ogen).
13. Hydroxyprogesterone caproate (Delalutin).
14. Micronor Nor-Q.D. (Ovrette).
15. Neomycin.

REVIEW QUESTIONS

1. d.	2. b.	3. a.	4. a.	5. d.
6. c.	7. a.	8. b.	9. a.	10. d.

Chapter 29

CIRCLE THE CORRECT ANSWER

1. increase.
2. increases, decreases.
3. increased.
4. decreases.
5. increase.
6. increase.
7. decrease.
8. increase.
9. decreased.
10. increase.
11. increases.
12. increase.
13. increase.
14. increase.
15. increase.
16. decrease.
17. increase.
18. increase.
19. increase.
20. increase.
21. increase.

CROSSWORD PUZZLE

ACROSS

2. Insulin.
3. Electrolyte.
5. Epiphyseal.
6. Delatestryl.
7. Baldness.
8. Durabolin.
9. Dependence.

DOWN

1. Danazol.
3. Exogenous.
4. Testosterone.

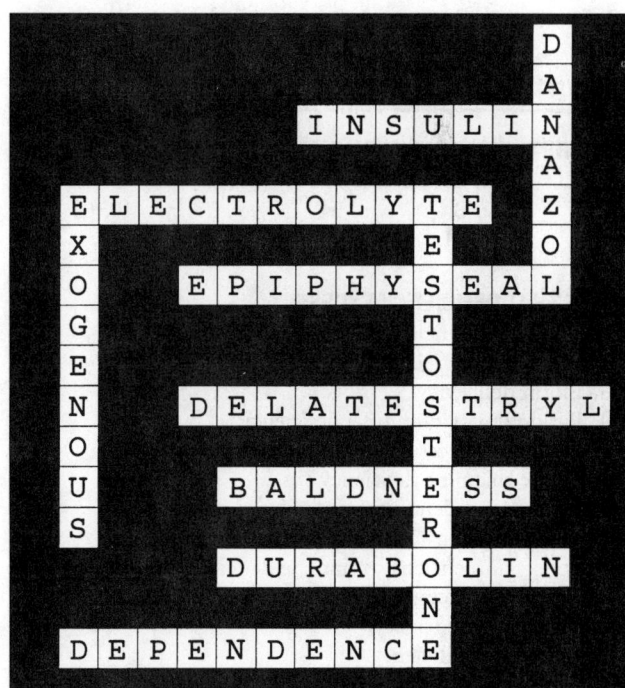

REVIEW QUESTIONS

1. b.	2. a.	3. c.	4. d.	5. a.
6. d.	7. d.	8. b.	9. a.	10. b.

Chapter 30

FILL IN THE BLANKS
1. P.   2. W.   3. P.   4. C & F.   5. W.

TRUE OR FALSE
1. F.   2. T.   3. F.   4. T.   5. F.
6. T.   7. F.   8. F.   9. T.   10. F.
11. F.   12. F.

MATCHING EXERCISE
1. C.   2. B.   3. F.   4. G.   5. E.
6. A.   7. D.   8. J.   9. I.   10. H.
11. K   12. L

FILL IN THE BLANKS
1. D_5W, water, normal saline.
2. 20%, 50%, hypertonic.
3. 550.
4. water.
5. hypertonic, increase.
6. protein, calories.
7. essential fatty acids, centrally, peripherally.
8. tube placement.
9. 500 mL.
10. 500–1000 mL.

REVIEW QUESTIONS
1. d.   2. a.   3. c.   4. c.   5. c.
6. c.   7. c.   8. d.   9. a.   10. a.

Chapter 31

MATCHING EXERCISE (TERMS AND CONCEPTS)
1. D.   2. F.   3. H.   4. J.   5. L.
6. A.   7. B.   8. E.   9. I.   10. C.
11. G.   12. M.   13. K.

NAME THAT DEFICIENCY/EXCESS
1. Vitamin A deficiency.
2. Vitamin K deficiency.
3. Biotin deficiency.
4. Pyridoxine (vitamin B_6) deficiency.
5. Vitamin C excess, vitamin A deficiency.
6. Severe thiamine deficiency.
7. Vitamin B_{12} deficiency.
8. Severe vitamin C deficiency.
9. Folic acid deficiency, thiamine deficiency.
10. Vitamin A excess.
11. Vitamin C deficiency.
12. Riboflavin deficiency.
13. Niacin deficiency.
14. Vitamin C excess.
15. Vitamin B_{12} deficiency.
16. Vitamin B_{12} deficiency.
17. Vitamin K deficiency.
18. Vitamin A excess.
19. Folic acid deficiency, thiamine deficiency.
20. Vitamin C deficiency.

REVIEW QUESTIONS
1. a.   2. b.   3. d.   4. b.   5. d.
6. d.   7. d.   8. a.   9. c.   10. d.

Chapter 32

MATCHING EXERCISE (TERMS AND CONCEPTS)
1. G.   2. F.   3. D.   4. H.   5. M.
6. I.   7. A.   8. K.   9. B.   10. P.
11. C.   12. E.   13. J.   14. L.   15. O.
16. N.

NAME THAT IMBALANCE
1. Hyperkalemia.
2. Zinc deficiency.
3. Hypernatremia.
4. Hypochloremia, hypokalemia.
5. Hyperkalemia.
6. Chromium deficiency.
7. Hypokalemia.
8. Hypocupremia.
9. Hyponatremia, hypomagnesemia, hypochloremia.
10. Hypermagnesemia, hypernatremia.
11. Hypernatremia.
12. Iron deficiency.
13. Hyponatremia.
14. Hypermagnesemia.
15. Hypokalemia.
16. Hyperchloremia.
17. Hypochloremia, hypocalcemia.
18. Hyperkalemia.
19. Hypomagnesemia.
20. Hypermagnesemia.

REVIEW QUESTIONS
1. b.   2. b.   3. d.   4. c.   5. b.
6. b.   7. a.   8. c.   9. c.   10. d.

Chapter 33

FILL IN THE BLANKS
1. a. bacteria.
   b. viruses.
   c. fungi.
2. occupying space and consuming nutrients.
3. superinfection, other hosts.
4. a. breaks in skin.
   b. impaired blood supply.
   c. neutropenia.
   d. malnutrition.
   e. poor hygiene.
   f. suppression of normal flora.
   g. suppression of immune system.
   h. diabetes mellitus.
   i. advanced age.
5. nosocomial.
6. antibacterials, antivirals, antifungals.
7. bactericidal.
8. bacteriostatic.
9. 7–10.
10. reduced, creatinine.

11. aminoglycosides.
12. clindamycin, erythromycin, cefaperazone, chloramphenicol.
13. a. hypersensitivity.
    b. superinfection.
    c. phlebitis.
    d. nausea and vomiting.
    e. diarrhea.
    f. nephrotoxicity.
    g. neurotoxicity.
    h. bleeding.
14. a. recurrence of symptoms.
    b. new localized signs and symptoms.
    c. stomatitis.
    d. pseudomembranous colitis.

REVIEW QUESTIONS

1. b.   2. a.   3. c.   4. c.   5. d.
6. d.   7. c.   8. d.   9. b.   10. c.

Chapter 34

FILL IN THE BLANKS

1. a. streptococcal pharyngitis.
   b. pneumococcal pneumonia.
   c. gonorrhea.
   d. syphilis.
2. respiratory, gastrointestinal, urinary.
3. cloxacillin, dicloxacillin, nafcillin, oxacillin.
4. ampicillin.
5. urinary tract, biliary tract, respiratory, ear.
6. ampicillin, sulbactam.
7. carbenicillin, ticarcillin, mezlocillin, piperacillin.
8. aminoglycoside.
9. gram-positive, gram-negative.
10. first-, second-, third-, fourth-.
11. a. respiratory tract.
    b. skin.
    c. soft tissue.
    d. joints.
    e. urinary tract.
    f. bloodstream.
12. meropenem (Merrem).

CROSSWORD PUZZLE

ACROSS

1. Penicillin.
8. Renal.
9. Cerebrospinal.
10. Cefazolin.
11. Augmentin.

DOWN

2. Ceftriaxone.
3. Prosthetic.
4. Mezlocillin.
5. Tetracyclines.
6. Cefoperazone.
7. Cephalexin.

REVIEW QUESTIONS

1. c.   2. b.   3. d.   4. d.   5. b.
6. c.   7. d.   8. d.   9. d.   10. a.

Chapter 35

FILL IN THE BLANKS

1. gram-negative.
2. urinary tract.
3. serious, life-threatening.
4. resistant to other drugs.
5. intestinal bacteria, ammonia.
6. a. check renal function studies.
   b. assess for hearing impairment.
   c. aminoglycosides to increase risk of nephrotoxicity.
7. serum drug levels, renal function studies, at least 2000–3000 mL.
8. age, weight, renal function, serum levels.
9. impaired renal function, inadequate fluid intake, prolonged exposure to sunlight.
10. a. children under 18.
    b. pregnant or lactating females.
    c. those who have had a hypersensitive reaction.
11. 30–60, trough, 10–12, 2.
12. 2–4.
13. diuretics.

REVIEW QUESTIONS

1. b.   2. d.   3. a.   4. b.   5. a.
6. a.   7. b.   8. c.   9. d.   10. d.

Chapter 36

FILL IN THE BLANKS

1. gram-positive, gram-negative, rickettsiae, mycoplasmas, protozoa, spirochetes.
2. urine, feces.
3. a. cholera.
   b. granuloma inguinale.
   c. chancroid.
   d. Rocky Mountain spotted fever.
   e. psittacosis.
   f. typhus.
   g. trachoma.
4. Demeclocycline, chronic.
5. mottling of tooth enamel, interfere with bone growth.
6. late pregnancy, lactation, children under 2 months.
7. allergic to salicylates, intestinal, urinary tract obstruction.
8. crystalluria.
9. acidic, ascorbic acid.
10. sunlight, sunlamps, tanning beds.
11. 1 hour before meals.
12. metallic ions.
13. severe nausea, vomiting, diarrhea, furry tongue, skin rash, perineal.
14. inhibit, kill.
15. (Macrodantin), acute, chronic, recurrent.
16. dye, dysuria, burning, frequency, urgency.
17. alkalinizing agents, methenamine compounds, salicylates.

CROSSWORD PUZZLE

ACROSS

4. Demeclocycline.
5. Bactrim.
6. Silvadene.

DOWN

1. Gantrisin.
2. Azulfidine.
3. Sulfamylon.

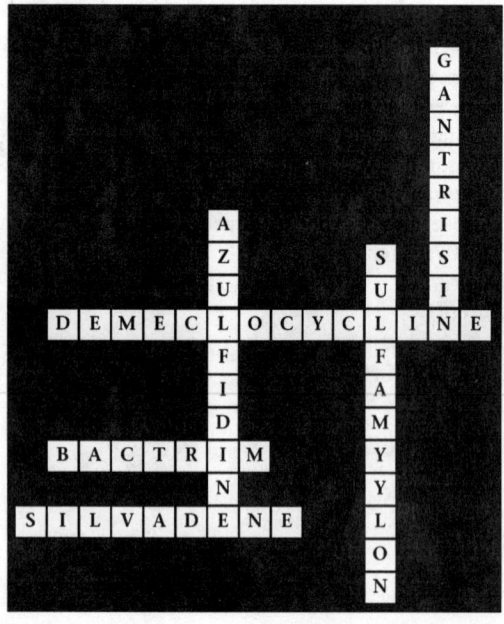

REVIEW QUESTIONS

1. a.	2. d.	3. c.	4. d.	5. d.
6. a.	7. b.	8. d.	9. c.	10. a.

Chapter 37

FILL IN THE BLANKS

1. diarrhea.
2. penicillin.
3. chlamydia trachomatis.
4. clarithromycin.
5. bile.
6. bacteria.
7. opportunistic.
8. typhoid.
9. erythromycin.
10. respiratory.
11. spectinomycin.
12. vancomycin.
13. macrolides.

A N T I B A C T E R I A L

REVIEW QUESTIONS

1. a.	2. a.	3. d.	4. b.	5. c.
6. d.	7. b.	8. b.	9. c.	10. d.

Chapter 38

FILL IN THE BLANKS

1. 6.
2. INH, rifampin, pyrazinamide, ethambutol, streptomycin.
3. skin test.
4. pyrazinamide, ofloxacin.
5. body weight.
6. metabolism, half-life, therapeutic effect.
7. para-aminosalicylic (PAS), capreomycin (Capastat), cycloserine (Seromycin), ethionamide (Trecator SC)
8. a. GI problems.
   b. Yellow sclera, dark urine, clay-colored stools.
   c. Changes in hearing or vision.
   d. Numbness or tingling.
   e. Dizziness, drowsiness.
   f. Skin rash or fever.

MATCHING EXERCISE

1. E.	2. A.	3. F.	4. B.	5. D.
6. C.				

IDENTIFY THE TREATMENT

1. A for INH.
2. A for rifampin; C for ethambutol and pyrazinamide.
3. C for pyrazinamide and ofloxacin.
4. C for INH, rifampin, and pyrazinamide.
5. C for INH, rifampin, and pyrazinamide; C* for ethambutol and streptomycin; √ for ofloxacin, amikacin, and ciprofloxacin.
6. C for INH, rifampin, and ethambutol.

REVIEW QUESTIONS

1. d.	2. a.	3. b.	4. d.	5. c.
6. d.	7. a.	8. d.	9. c.	10. d.

Chapter 39

TRUE OR FALSE

1. F.	2. F.	3. T.	4. F.	5. T.
6. T.	7. F.	8. T.	9. F.	10. T.
11. F.	12. T.	13. F.	14. T.	15. T.

MATCHING EXERCISE

1. E.	2. A.	3. D.	4. B.	5. C.	6. F.

REVIEW QUESTIONS

1. a.	2. b.	3. b.	4. a.	5. d.
6. d.	7. a.	8. b.	9. c.	10. a.

Chapter 40

MATCHING EXERCISE

1. A.	2. G.	3. F.	4. J.	5. I.
6. C.	7. H.	8. E.	9. B.	10. D.
11. O.	12. K.	13. M.	14. N.	15. Q.
16. S.	17. R.	18. T.	19. P	20. L

FILL IN THE BLANKS

1. inhalation, oral ingestion, implantation.
2. topically.
3. histoplasmosis.
4. candidal.
5. Amphotericin B (Fungizone).

REVIEW QUESTIONS

1. b.	2. a.	3. a.	4. b.	5. b.
6. d.	7. d.	8. b.	9. a.	10. b.

Chapter 41

TRUE OR FALSE

1. T.	2. T.	3. T.	4. F.	5. F.
6. T.	7. T.	8. F.	9. T.	10. F.
11. T.	12. T.	13. T.	14. T.	15. T.
16. T.				

REVIEW QUESTIONS

1. c.	2. a.	3. c.	4. c.	5. b.
6. a.	7. c.	8. b.	9. c.	10. d.

Chapter 42

MATCHING EXERCISE

1. D.	2. A.	3. H.	4. J.	5. B.
6. C.	7. E.	8. O.	9. L.	10. F.
11. N.	12. I.	13. G.	14. K.	15. M.

REVIEW QUESTIONS

1. c.	2. d.	3. c.	4. a.	5. a.
6. a.	7. a.	8. b.	9. a.	10. d.

Chapter 43

FILL IN THE BLANKS

1. antigen, antibody formation.
2. antibodies.
3. killed, attentuated.
4. toxicity while retaining antigenic properties.
5. diphtheria, hepatitis B, tetanus, pertussis, rubeola, rubella, mumps, poliomyelitis.
6. pregnancy, febrile illness, immunosuppressive drug therapy, immunodeficiency states.
7. epinephrine.
8. tenderness, redness, Tylenol.
9. paralysis (Guillain-Barré syndrome).
10. influenza vaccine, pneumococcal.

EXERCISE ON IMMUNIZATION

1. SC.	2. IM.	3. PO.	4. IM.

REVIEW QUESTIONS

1. d.	2. c.	3. a.	4. a.	5. d.
6. b.	7. c.	8. a.	9. a.	10. b.

Chapter 44

MATCHING EXERCISE

1. B.	2. J.	3. F.	4. D.	5. I.
6. G.	7. E.	8. A.	9. K.	10. H.

TRUE OR FALSE

1. T.	2. F.	3. F.	4. T.	5. T.

CROSSWORD PUZZLE

ACROSS

1. Aldesleukin.
3. Interferon.
4. Neutrophil.
6. Condylomata.
8. Filgrastim.
9. Leukopenia.

DOWN

2. Sargramostim.
5. BCG.
7. Solid.

REVIEW QUESTIONS

1. a.	2. a.	3. a.	4. c.	5. c.
6. c.	7. d.	8. d.	9. c.	10. c.

Schedule for Immunization of Infants and Children

Place an x in the table to identify the appropriate timing(s) for immunizations, based upon recommendations from the Advisory Committee on Immunization Practices (ACIP), the American Academy of Pediatrics (AAP), and the American Academy of Family Physicians (AAFP).

	Birth	1 mo	2 mo	4 mo	6 mo	10-12 mo	15 mo	18 mo	4-6 yr	Every 11-12 yr	10 yr	14-16
Polio (IPV)			X	X	←——————————→				X			
Diphtheria-tetanus-pertussis (DTP)			X	X	X			x	X			
Diphtheria-tetanus (DT)											X	X
Measles-mumps-rubella (MMR)			X			←——————————→						
Haemophilus influenza Type B (Hib)			X	X	X	←——————————→						
Hepatitis B (HBV)	X	X——X	X		X	X						
Varicella zoster (Var) chicken pox						←——————————→				X		

(Adapted by Rachel Hofstetter)
Based upon recommendations from the Advisory Committee on Immunization Practices (ACIP), the American Academy of Pediatrics (AAP), and the American Academy of Family Physicians (AAFP). Arrows indicate that immunization should be done within the marked span of time.

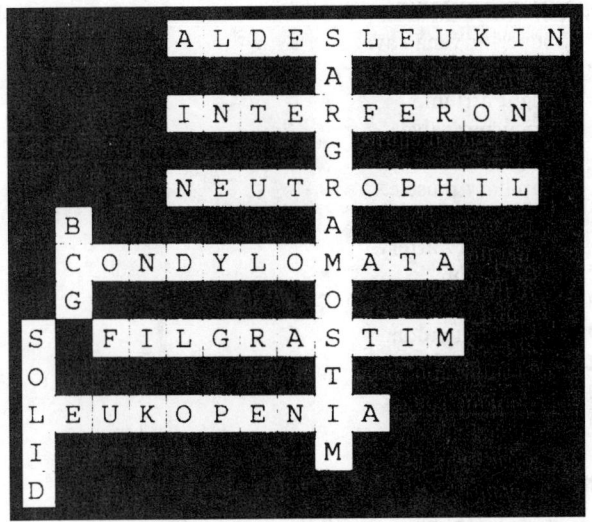

Chapter 45

TRUE OR FALSE
1. T.	2. F.	3. F.	4. F.	5. T.
6. T.	7. T.	8. F.	9. F.	10. F.
11. T.	12. T.	13. F.	14. F.	15. T.

REVIEW QUESTIONS
1. a.	2. b.	3. a.	4. a.	5. c.
6. b.	7. a.	8. d.	9. c.	10. b.

Chapter 46

MATCHING EXERCISE (TERMS AND CONCEPTS)
1. D.	2. E.	3. C.	4. K.	5. F.
6. B.	7. M.	8. I.	9. L.	10. O.

RESPIRATORY SYSTEM DIAGRAM
1. B.	2. A.	3. D.	4. C.	5. G.
6. E.	7. F.			

REVIEW QUESTIONS
1. d.	2. b.	3. c.	4. a.	5. d.
6. b.	7. c.	8. a.	9. a.	10. c.

Chapter 47

MATCHING EXERCISE
1. B.	2. C.	3. D.	4. A.

FILL IN THE BLANKS
1. a. respiratory infections.
   b. odors.
   c. smoke.
   d. cold air.
   e. exercise.
   f. tartrazine.
   g. fumes.

h. drugs.
2. (Adrenalin), acute attack of bronchospasm, 5 minutes.
3. (Proventil), orally, inhalation.
4. (Atrovent), 15, cough, nervousness, nausea, GI upset, headache, dizziness.
5. (Beclovent), (Vanceril), (Azmacort), inhalation.
6. (Intal), prophylaxis of acute asthma attacks in clients with chronic asthma.
7. confusion, restlessness, anxiety, increased BP, increased pulse.
8. coughing, deep breathing, percussion, postural drainage.
9. bronchodilator.
10. fungal infection of the mouth and throat.

TRUE OR FALSE
1. F.	2. T.	3. T.	4. F.	5. F.
6. T.				

REVIEW QUESTIONS
1. d.	2. d.	3. d.	4. d.	5. d.
6. b.	7. d.	8. b.	9. c.	10. a.

Chapter 48

MATCHING EXERCISE (TERMS AND CONCEPTS)
1. B.	2. C.	3. G.	4. E.	5. A.
6. F.	7. H.	8. J.	9. I.	10. D.
11. L.	12. N.			

DEFINITIONS
1. Anaphylaxis is characterized by cardiovascular collapse and respiratory distress.
2. Serum sickness is a delayed hypersensitivity reaction often caused by drugs.
3. Hypersensitivity occurs several hours or days after exposure to an antigen.
4. Anaphylactoid reaction is not an antigen antibody reaction and may occur on the first exposure to the causative agent.

REVIEW QUESTIONS
1. c.	2. a.	3. d.	4. c.	5. b.
6. d.	7. a.	8. d.	9. d.	10. b.

Chapter 49

FILL IN THE BLANKS
1. common cold, sinusitis, nasal congestion, cough, secretions.
2. profuse discharge from the nose.
3. cough.
4. immobility, cigarette smoking, surgical procedures.
5. rest and sleep.
6. acetylcysteine (Mucomyst).
7. antihistamines, nasal decongestants, analgesics, antitussives, expectorants.
8. rebound nasal congestion.

9. increase.
10. nausea, vomiting, constipation, dizziness, drowsiness, pruritus, drug dependence.
11. arrhythmias, hypertension.
12. blow his or her nose.
13. 20–30 minutes before feeding.
14. 30 minutes.
15. 2000–3000 mL.

CROSSWORD PUZZLE

ACROSS
1. Sudafed.
5. Dextromethorphan.
9. Nasal.

DOWN
2. Acetylcysteine.
3. Acetaminophen.
4. Rhinitis.
5. Dimetapp.
6. Otrivin.
7. Robitussin.
8. Antitussives.

REVIEW QUESTIONS
1. c.	2. d.	3. a.	4. d.	5. b.
6. c.	7. a.	8. c.	9. c.	

Chapter 50

MATCHING EXERCISE (TERMS AND CONCEPTS)
1. C.	2. A.	3. F.	4. G.	5. J.
6. K.	7. L.	8. N.	9. H.	10. M.

FILL IN THE BLANKS
1. Superior vena cava.
2. Coronary arteries.
3. Right atrium.
4. Tricuspid valve.
5. Inferior vena cava.
6. Papillary muscle.
7. Aorta.
8. Pulmonary artery.
9. Left atrium.
10. Mitral valve.
11. Chordae tendon.
12. Left ventricle.
13. Septum.
14. Right ventricle.

REVIEW QUESTIONS
1. a.	2. b.	3. b.	4. b.	5. d.
6. c.	7. c.	8. d.	9. a.	10. c.

Chapter 51

FILL IN THE BLANKS
1. increases, increases, vasoconstriction, increases, increases, ventricular hypertrophy.
2. preload.
3. increase, empty more completely.
4. fibrillation, flutter.
5. 0.75–1 mg.
6. 0.1 mg.
7. 0.057 mg.
8. (Inocor), short-term.
9. digoxin toxicity.
10. a. large doses.
    b. rapid digitalization.
    c. impaired renal function.
    d. age extremes.
    e. electrolyte imbalances.
    f. hypoxia.
    g. hypothyroidism.
    h. concurrent treatment with other drugs.
11. a. 1. atherosclerosis
       2. hypertension
       3. coronary artery disease
       4. myocardial infarction
       5. cardiac arrhythmias
       6. cardiac valvular disease
    b. 1. severe infection
       2. hyperthyroidism
       3. pulmonary disease
    c. 1. excessive fluids
       2. advanced age
12. diuretics, cardiotonic-inotropic agents, vasodilators.

MATCHING EXERCISE (TERMS AND CONCEPTS)
1. F.	2. H.	3. K.	4. A.	5. E.
6. G.	7. M.	8. D.	9. J.	10. I.
11. L.	12. N	13. C.	14. B.	

REVIEW QUESTIONS
1. b.   2. c.   3. b.   4. d.   5. b.
6. c.   7. c.   8. a.   9. a.   10. a.

Chapter 52

MATCHING EXERCISE (TERMS AND CONCEPTS)
1. B.   2. A.   3. F.   4. G.   5. J.
6. M.   7. I.   8. E.   9. D.   10. C.
11. H.   12. L.   13. F.

CROSSWORD PUZZLE

ACROSS
9. Digoxin.
10. Disopyramide.

DOWN
1. Quinidine.
2. Propranolol.
3. Pronestyl.
4. Lidocaine.
5. Moricizine.
6. Atropine.
7. Brevibloc.
8. Verapamil.

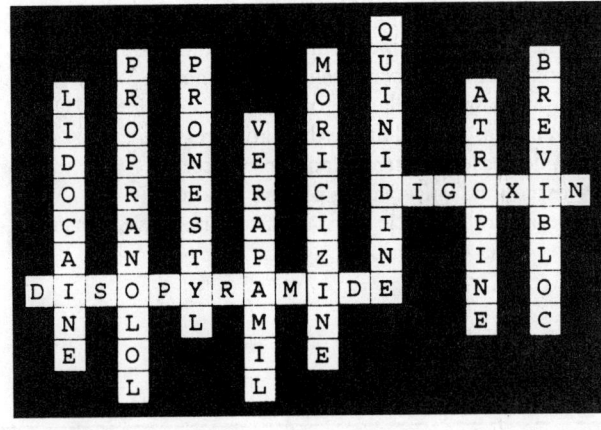

CARDIAC ELECTROPHYSIOLOGY EXERCISE—PART I: DIAGRAM COMPLETION
1. Left atrium.
2. Left ventricle.
3. Left bundle branch.
4. Purkinje fibers.
5. Right bundle branch.
6. Bundle of His.
7. Right ventricle.
8. AV node.
9. Right atrium.
10. SA node.

CARDIAC ELECTROPHYSIOLOGY EXERCISE—PART II: DRUG EFFECTS ON CARDIAC PHYSIOLOGY
1. 7, right ventricle; 2, left ventricle.
2. 10, SA node; 8, AV node.
3. 8, AV node; 6, bundle of His; 5, right bundle branch; 7, right ventricle; 3, left bundle branch; 2, left ventricle.
4. 10, SA node; 8, AV node.

DYSRHYTHMIA ANALYSIS
1. Supraventricular tachycardia, adenosine (Adenocard).
2. Atrial fibrillation, digoxin (Lanoxin).
3. Sinus bradycardia, atropine.
4. Premature ventricular contractions, lidocaine (Xylocaine).

REVIEW QUESTIONS
1. b.   2. a.   3. c.   4. b.   5. b.
6. b.   7. c.   8. b.   9. a.   10. b.

Chapter 53

FILL IN THE BLANKS
1. venous pressure, venous return to the heart, blood volume, blood pressure (preload), cardiac workload, oxygen demand, flow to the myocardium, peripheral resistance.
2. heart rate, myocardial contractility, blood pressure, myocardial workload, oxygen demand.
3. hypotension, bradycardia, bronchospasm, congestive heart failure.
4. coronary, peripheral arteries, myocardial contractility.
5. heavy meals, cigarette smoking, strenuous exercise.
6. diet, adequate rest.
7. 5, three, see their physician.
8. hypotension, dizziness, headaches.
9. a. x.
   b. x.
   c.
   d. x.
   e.
   f.
   g. x.
   h. x.
10. avoid strenuous exercise, assume a supine position.

MATCHING EXERCISE (TERMS AND CONCEPTS)
1. E.   2. B.   3. G.   4. A.   5. I.
6. H.   7. K.   8. C.   9. F.   10. L.

FILL IN THE BLANKS (EFFECTS OF NITROGLYCERIN)
1. arterioles.
2. veins.
3. peripheral resistance.
4. venous return.
5. afterload (blood pressure).
6. preload (venous return).
7. workload.
8. oxygen demand.

REVIEW QUESTIONS
1. d.   2. d.   3. b.   4. b.   5. c.
6. c.   7. a.   8. a.   9. d.   10. c.

Chapter 54

TRUE OR FALSE
1. F.   2. F.   3. T.   4. T.   5. F.
6. T.   7. F.   8. T.   9. F.   10. T.

FILL IN THE BLANKS
1. decreased, decreased, decreased.
2. peripheral vascular resistance.
3. myocardial contractility, heart rate.
4. 90/60, 50 mL/hr.
5. phentolamine (Regitine).
6. hypovolemic, cardiogenic, anaphylactic, neurogenic, septic.

REVIEW QUESTIONS
1. b.   2. a.   3. a.   4. d.   5. b.
6. b.   7. d.   8. a.   9. a.   10. b.

Chapter 55

MATCHING EXERCISE (TERMS AND CONCEPTS)
1. E.   2. A.   3. F.   4. B.   5. C.
6. D.   7. G.

NAME THAT DRUG
1. Calcium channel blockers.
2. Hydralazine (Apresoline).
3. Sodium nitroprusside (Nipride).
4. Hydrochlorothiazide (Hydrodiuril).
5. Beta blockers.

6. Beta blockers, calcium channel blockers.
7. Vasodilators.
8. Clonidine (Catapres).
9. Diet and exercise.
10. Angiotensin II receptor antagonists, ACE inhibitors plus loop diuretics.
11. Thiazide diuretics.
12. Reserpine (Serpasil).
13. Clonidine (Catapres), guanabenz (Wytensin).
14. Enalapril (Vasotec), lisinopril (Zestril).
15. Alpha blockers, direct vasodilators.
16. Nonselective beta blockers, propranolol (Inderal).

FILL IN THE BLANKS
See chart below.

REVIEW QUESTIONS
1. a.   2. d.   3. b.   4. b.   5. a.
6. d.   7. c.   8. d.   9. c.   10. c.

Chapter 56

FILL IN THE BLANKS
1. glomerular filtration, tubular reabsorption, tubular secretion.
2. 400 mL, normal amounts, metabolic endproducts.
3. proximal tubule.
4. Antidiuretic hormone, water.
5. Aldosterone, sodium, potassium.
6. uric acid, creatinine, hydrogen ions, ammonia.
7. potassium ions, hydrogen ions, ammonia.
8. a. increased capillary permeability.
    b. increased capillary hydrostatic pressure.
    c. decreased plasma osmotic pressure.
9. tissue fluids, decreasing plasma volume.
10. peripheral vascular resistance, sodium, have a vasodilating effect on arterioles.

CARDIOVASCULAR INDICATIONS FOR USE

	Angina Pectoris	Hypertension	Arrhythmias	Heart Failure	MI
Losartan (Cozaar)		X		X	
Diltiazem (Cardizem)	X	X*			
Nifedipine (Adalat, Procardia)	X	X*			
Verapamil (Calan, Isoptin)	X	X	X		
Captopril (Capoten)		X		X	
Propranolol (Inderal)	X	X	X		X
Metoprolol (Lopressor)		X			X
Esmolol (Brevibloc)			X		

* Only the sustained release formulations (diltiazem SR and nifedipine SR) are approved for treatment of hypertension.

11. Thiazide diuretics, 2.
12. sodium, potassium, Hyperkalemia.
13. solute load (osmotic pressure), water, bloodstream, Mannitol.
14. electrolytes, uric acid, blood glucose, creatinine, BUN.
15. blood pressure, weight, urine output, edematous extremities.
16. digoxin toxicity, diuretic-induced hypokalemia.
17. 3.5–5.0 mEq/L.
18. a. giving supplemental potassium.
    b. giving a potassium-sparing diuretic.
    c. increasing potassium intake.
    d. using salt substitutes.
    e. restricting sodium.
19. a. ECG changes.
    b. dysrhythmias.
    c. hypotension.
    d. weak shallow respiration.
    e. anorexia.
    f. nausea, vomiting.
    g. paralytic ileus.
    h. skeletal muscle weakness.
    i. confusion, disorientation.

TRUE OR FALSE

1. F.	2. T.	3. T.	4. F.	5. F.
6. F.	7. F.	8. F.	9. T.	10. F.

FILL IN THE BLANKS: THE NEPHRON

1. Efferent arteriole.
2. Afferent arteriole.
3. Bowman's capsule.
4. Glomerulus.
5. Distal tubule.
6. Proximal tubule.
7. Collecting tubule.
8. Descending limb of loop of Henle.
9. Ascending limb of loop of Henle.
10. Loop of Henle.

REVIEW QUESTIONS

1. c.	2. c.	3. d.	4. a.	5. b.
6. a.	7. b.	8. c.	9. b.	10. c.

Chapter 57

FILL IN THE BLANKS

1. Increase.
2. Increase.
3. Increase.
4. Decrease.
5. Increase.
6. Decrease.
7. Increase.
8. Increase.
9. Decrease.
10. Decrease.

DRUG INDICATIONS AND ACTIONS: HEPARIN

1. Acute thromboembolic problems, prophylaxis for clients at risk following administration of thrombolytic agents.
2. Rapid, within minutes.
3. Short.
4. IV, SC.
5. Activated partial thromboplastin time (APTT).
6. Protamine sulfate.

DRUG INDICATIONS AND ACTIONS: COUMADIN

1. Long–term treatment for prevention of clot formation.
2. Delayed 2–5 days.
3. 2–5 days after discontinuation.
4. PO.
5. Prothrombin time (PT) and International Normalized Ratio (INR).
6. Vitamin K.

DRUG INDICATIONS AND ACTIONS: RETAVASE

1. To dissolve thrombi and limit tissue damage.
2. Immediate.
3. Minutes after discontinuation.
4. IV.
5. Thrombin time (TT), activated partial thromboplastin time (APTT), prothrombin time (PT).
6. Discontinue infusion, whole blood packed cells or fresh frozen plasma, Amicar.

REVIEW QUESTIONS

1. b.	2. b.	3. b.	4. c.	5. d.
6. c.	7. c.	8. a.	9. c.	10. c.

Chapter 58

MATCHING EXERCISE (TERMS AND CONCEPTS)

1. C.	2. B.	3. D.	4. A.

REVIEW QUESTIONS

1. b.	2. a.	3. a.	4. b.	5. b.
6. c.	7. d.	8. b.	9. c.	10. d.

CHAPTER 58 FILL IN THE BLANKS

Treatment	Hyperlipidemia					
	I	IIa	IIb	III	IV	V
Cholestyramine (Questran)		X				
Pravastatin (Pravachol)		X	X			
Gemfibrozil (Lopid)					X	X
Nicotinic acid (Niacin)		X	X	X	X	X
Atorvastatin (Lipitor)		X	X			
Lovastatin (Mevacor)		X	X			
Diet modification	X	X	X	X	X	X
Exercise	X	X	X	X	X	X

Chapter 59

MATCHING EXERCISE (TERMS AND CONCEPTS)
1. D. 2. E. 3. F. 4. G. 5. A.
6. I. 7. K. 8. B. 9. C. 10. M.
11. N. 12. O. 13. P. 14. Q. 15. R.

DIGESTIVE SYSTEM DIAGRAM
1. G. 2. C. 3. A. 4. B. 5. E.
6. D. 7. F.

REVIEW QUESTIONS
1. b. 2. a. 3. c. 4. b. 5. c.
6. d. 7. b. 8. b. 9. c. 10. d.

Chapter 60

MATCHING EXERCISE (TERMS AND CONCEPTS)
1. B. 2. C. 3. D. 4. A. 5. E.
6. F. 7. I. 8. H. 9. G. 10. J.

TRUE OR FALSE
1. T. 2. F. 3. F. 4. F. 5. F.
6. F. 7. T. 8. F. 9. T. 10. T.

FILL IN THE BLANKS
1. esophogeal reflux, GI bleeding, esophagitis, stress ulcers, gastritis, heart burn.
2. gastric acid.
3. amount, acidity, pepsin content.
4. potent, drug interactions.
5. Pepcid, Axid, mental confusion, gynecomastia.
6. Cytotec, GI bleeding.
7. Carafate, ulcer, coating, healing.
8. a. cigarette smoking.
   b. stress.
   c. genetic influences.
   d. sex.
   e. drug therapy.

MATCHING EXERCISE
1. D. 2. F. 3. C. 4. G. 5. E.
6. B. 7. H. 8. A.

CROSSWORD PUZZLE

ACROSS
1. Misoprostol.
4. Sodium.
9. Calcium.
10. Hypersecretion.

DOWN
2. Prostaglandins.
3. Palatability.
5. Cimetidine.
6. Aluminum.
7. Omeprazole.
8. Sucralfate.

REVIEW QUESTIONS

1. b.	2. c.	3. c.	4. c.	5. b.
6. b.	7. a.	8. b.	9. d.	10. a.

Chapter 61

MATCHING EXERCISE (TERMS AND CONCEPTS)

1. F.	2. E.	3. A.	4. D.	5. G.
6. B.	7. H.	8. C.	9. I.	10. J.
11. L.	12. N.	13. O.	14. Q.	15. P.

DEFINITIONS

1. Laxatives that decrease the surface tension of the fecal mass and allow water to penetrate.
2. The elimination of feces from the colon.
3. Infrequent, painful explusion of dry, hard stool.

REVIEW QUESTIONS

1. a.	2. d.	3. c.	4. a.	5. b.
6. a.	7. c.	8. a.	9. a.	10. c.

Chapter 62

TRUE OR FALSE

1. F.	2. T.	3. T.	4. T.	5. F.
6. T.	7. T.	8. F.	9. T.	10. F.
11. T.	12. F.	13. F.	14. F.	15. T.

FILL IN THE BLANKS

1. a. intestinal infections.
   b. undigested/coarse/spiced foods.
   c. excessive use of laxatives.
   d. lack of digestive enzymes.
   e. inflammatory bowel disease.
   f. drug therapy.
   g. intestinal neoplasms.
   h. stress.
   i. hyperthyroidism.
   j. surgery.
   k. AIDS/HIV.
2. a. replacement fluids (tea, bouillon, Jell-o).
   b. restrict oral intake.
   c. rest.
   d. avoid foods that irritate the GI mucosa.

REVIEW QUESTIONS

1. b.	2. b.	3. a.	4. b.	5. c.
6. d.	7. c.	8. c.	9. b.	10. d.

Chapter 63

MATCHING EXERCISE (TERMS AND CONCEPTS)

1. J.	2. A.	3. I.	4. B.	5. C.
6. H.	7. D.	8. G.	9. E.	10. F.
11. O.	12. L.	13. N.	14. M.	15. P.
16. Q.	17. K.			

REVIEW QUESTIONS

1. b.	2. d.	3. c.	4. b.	5. c.
6. c.	7. a.	8. b.	9. b.	

Chapter 64

MATCHING EXERCISE (TERMS AND CONCEPTS)

1. D.	2. J.	3. A.	4. B.	5. H.
6. G.	7. F.	8. C.	9. E.	10. L.
11. K.	12. O.	13. M.	14. N.	

FILL IN THE BLANKS

1. tissue type, rate of growth, other characteristics.
2. hematologic, solid.
3. bone marrow.
4. lymphoid tissue.
5. epithelial, skin, mucous membrane, viscera.
6. connective, bone, cartilage, fibrous tissue, fat, blood vessels.
7. a. alkylating agents
   b. antimetabolites
   c. antitumor antibiotics
   d. plant alkaloids.
   e. hormones and hormone inhibitors.
   f. miscellaneous.

FILL IN THE BLANKS: CELL CYCLE

1. Mitosis occurs.
2. Resting phase.
3. RNA and enzymes required for the production of DNA are developed.
4. DNA is synthesized for chromosomes.
5. RNA is synthesized and the mitotic spindle is formed.
   a. taxanes or taxoids.
   b. vinca alkaloids.
   c. steroids.
   d. alkylating agents.
   e. antibiotics.
   f. nitrosureas.
   g. antimetabolites.
   h. podophyllotoxins.

REVIEW QUESTIONS

1. a.	2. a.	3. d.	4. c.	5. b.
6. b.	7. d.	8. a.	9. c.	10. d.

Chapter 65

MATCHING EXERCISE (TERMS AND CONCEPTS)

1. E.	2. D.	3. C.	4. B.	5. A.
6. J.	7. F.	8. G.	9. I.	10. H.
11. O.	12. N.	13. M.	14. L.	15. K.

FILL IN THE BLANKS

1. dilate the pupils.
2. inflammatory conditions.
3. decreases.
4. dye, diagnose.
5. increased intraocular pressure, four, constrict.
6. dilate, glaucoma.

Study Guide to Accompany Clinical Drug Therapy: Rationales for Nursing Practice, sixth edition, by Gail Ropelewski-Ryan.

7. weekly, glaucoma.
8. decreased production of aqueous humor, decreased ocular pressure.
9. irrigating the eyes with copious amounts of water as soon as possible.
10. trifluridine (Viroptic).

ANATOMY OF THE EYE

1. Iris.
2. Cornea.
3. Pupil.
4. Anterior chamber.
5. Lens.
6. Vitreous body.
7. Retina.
8. Choroid.
9. Sclera.
10. Optic disc.
11. Optic nerve.

NAME THAT DRUG

1. Osmotic diuretics.
2. Miotics.
3. Anticholinergics.
4. Carbonic anhydrase inhibitors.
5. Beta blockers.

DRUG CLASSIFICATION

1. Dipivefrin (Propine); *use*: glaucoma examinations, uveitis, pre- and post-op mydriasis, local hemostasis.
2. Timolol maleate (Timoptic); *use*: glaucoma.
3. Pilocarpine (Pilocar); *use*: glaucoma.
4. Demecarum bromide (Humorsol); *use*: glaucoma.
5. Atropine sulfate; *use*: examinations, pre- and post-op uveitis, secondary glaucoma.
6. Acetazolamide (Diamox); *use*: glaucoma, pre-op.
7. Glycerin (Osmoglyn); *use*: pre-op, acute glaucoma.
8. Apraclonidine (Iopidine); *use*: glaucoma, prevention of increased intraocular pressure after ocular surgery.
9. Proparacaine hydrochloride (Alcaine); *use*: local anesthetic.
10. Methylcellulose (Methulose); *use*: protect cornea during eye exams, keratitis, or wearing contact lenses.
11. Latanoprost (Xalatan); *use*: glaucoma.

REVIEW QUESTIONS

1. b.	2. a.	3. c.	4. a.	5. c.
6. a.	7. b.	8. d.	9. d.	10. d.

Chapter 66

MATCHING EXERCISE (TERMS AND CONCEPTS)

1. N.	2. A.	3. M.	4. B.	5. L.
6. C.	7. K.	8. D.	9. J.	10. E.
11. F.	12. I.	13. G.	14. H.	15. O.
16. T.	17. P.	18. S.	19. Q.	20. R.

DEFINE

1. flat spot
2. raised spot
3. small solid swelling
4. blister
5. pus containing lesions
6. redness

REVIEW QUESTIONS

1. a.	2. a.	3. d.	4. a.	5. a.
6. c.	7. a.	8. b.	9. c.	10. b.

Chapter 67

CHECKLIST: CONTRAINDICATED DRUGS

1.	2. ×	3.	4. ×	5. ×
6.	7.	8. ×	9.	10. ×
11. ×	12. ×	13. ×		

MATCHING EXERCISE: DRUGS AND INDICATIONS

1. F.	2. A.	3. E.	4. B.	5. C.
6. D.	7. K.	8. J.	9. I.	10. H.

FILL IN THE BLANKS: VASCULAR SYSTEM

1. increases.
2. 50, increase, increase.
3. increased.
4. anemia.
5. increase.
6. fall, decreased.
7. increased.
8. increased, decreased, decreased, prolonged.

REVIEW QUESTIONS

1. a.	2. c.	3. a.	4. d.	5. b.
6. a.	7. a.	8. a.	9. a.	10. b.

Appendix

1. 2 tablets.
2. 25 mL.
3. 10 mL.
4. 300 mg.
5. 6.7 mL.
6. 20 mL.
7. 83 mL/hr, 14 drops/min.
8. 125 mL/hr, 31 drops/min.
9. 30 drops/min.
10. 5 mL, 31 drops/min.
11. 500 mL.
12. 25 drops/min.
13. 0.3 mL.
14. 1.5 mL Demerol, 0.6 mL Atropine, 0.5 mL Vistaril; yes, these medications can be administered in the same syringe (total volume = 1.5 mL + 0.6 mL + 0.5 mL = 2.6 mL; can use one or two syringes).
15. 1.5 mL.
16. 12 mL.
17. 1000 U/hr.
18. 20 mg/hr.
19. 30 mL/hr.
20. 12 mL/hr.
21. 200 mcg/hr.
22. 40 mg/hr.
23. 0.33 mg/min.
24. 30 drops/min.
25. 48 mg/hr.
26. 0.5 mg/hr.
27. 12.5 mg/hr.
28. 12 U/hr.
29. 1 mg/min.
30. 25,000 U/min.